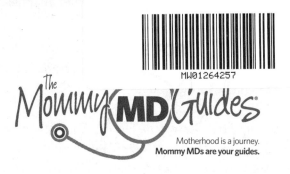

Motherhood is a journey.
Mommy MDs are your guides.

It is fascinating to find the real experiences of physician moms interposed with solid data about healthy pregnancy and delivery. *The Mommy MD Guide to Pregnancy and Birth* is an enjoyable and enlightening book that will "hold hands" with women through their pregnancies.

—*Joanna M. Cain, MD, Chace/Joukowsky Professor and chair, assistant dean of women's health at the Warren Alpert Medical School of Brown University, and obstetrician and gynecologist-in-chief at Women & Infants Hospital, both in Providence, RI*

∽

The Mommy MD Guide to Your Baby's First Year is fun, easy to read, and informative. I love that the advice from physicians is practical and based on experience, in addition to medical expertise.

Since it is a series of vignettes, it's easy to read and pick up in between other activities, which is ideal for busy people like me and new moms.

—*Jennifer Arnold, MD, a neonatologist and the medical director of the Pediatric Simulation Center at Texas*

Children's Hospital and an assistant professor at Baylor College of Medicine, both in Houston, and the star of TLC's The Little Couple

❧

The Mommy MD Guide to the Toddler Years is a great testament to the fact that no two kids or parents are exactly alike. I am always looking for new ideas for entertaining, disciplining, teaching, and loving on my kids because what worked with my first child doesn't always work with the other five! I love that this book accepts, appreciates, and addresses the fact that there isn't just one answer to any question or concern parents have with their children. For me, the more suggestions I can get, the better!

—*Casey Jones, a mom of a 9-year-old daughter and 4-year-old quintuplets and costar of* Quints by Surprise, *in Austin, TX*

❧

I found a quiet corner in the living room and flipped open *The Mommy MD Guide to Pregnancy and Birth*, about a topic I last experienced 10 years ago. The more I read, the more I kept thinking to myself, "I wish this book had been *around* 10 years ago." I would have devoured every word if I'd read it 20 years ago, as I plodded through my very first experience with the baffling world of pregnancy. This book really is different from every other pregnancy book I've read.

The Mommy MD Guide to Pregnancy and Birth has

advice from 60 doctors who are moms. Aside from the great medical advice, I was drawn to the anecdotal feeling of this book. As I read, I felt like I was sitting in the living room with these women as they shared their personal stories. I'm a person who loves to hear a good birth story, and I was really drawn to the personal nature of the advice. Instead of feeling like it was coming from a textbook, the advice feels like it's coming from a girlfriend who's just navigated the road herself. But it went beyond "just" a girlfriend's guide, because it was a girlfriend's guide times 60.

I highly recommend *The Mommy MD Guide to Pregnancy and Birth*. I have a feeling many dads wouldn't mind reading it either since it's not long chapters of information, but short snippets of advice, gathered in a very logical way.

I enjoyed the website that's hosted by the authors and look forward to the series this team is working on, covering the other stages of parenting, from newborn sleep issues to elementary school struggles. It's a great idea that was truly done right.

—*Judy Berna, a mom of four and writer for GeekMom.com*

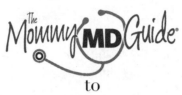

to

Twins,
Triplets,
and More

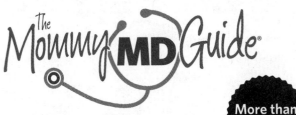

The Mommy MD Guide®

More than 200 tips!

to

Twins, Triplets, and More

Tips that 12 doctors who are also mothers
of multiples use to raise their own
twins, triplets, and more

by Sonal R. Patel, MD
and Heather Karpinsky

© 2018 by Momosa Publishing LLC

Printed in the United States of America

Cover design by Leanne Coppola
Interior design by Jennifer Giandomenico

Library of Congress information available upon request

ISBN 978-0-9994151-8-4

2 4 6 8 10 9 7 5 3 1 paperback

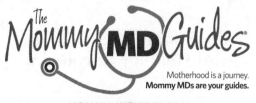

Motherhood is a journey.
Mommy MDs are your guides.

MOMMYMDGUIDES.COM

Contents

Introductions 13

Chapter 1: Pregnancy and Birth 17

Chapter 2: Feeding 40

Chapter 3: Diapering and Dressing 58

Chapter 4: Sleeping 73

Chapter 5: Coping with Health Challenges 89

Chapter 6: Staying Safe 100

Chapter 7: Fostering Personality 114

Chapter 8: Going to School and Work 127

Chapter 9: Outings, Day Trips, and Vacations 138

Index 159
Acknowledgments 169
About the Authors 173

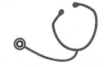

Introductions

Congratulations! You're either pregnant with twins or already in the midst of the beautiful chaos that is parenting multiples. Either way, it's an awesome adventure. I imagine you are filled with many emotions, including excitement, fear, and anxiety. You're not alone. We're about to offer you some wonderful suggestions and recommendations to help you deal with the emotional and physical demands of parenting multiples.

Parenting is one of the hardest things that I've ever had to do. Making it through medical school and residency were not easy feats, so that's really saying something. I'm not sure why no one tells you parenting will be so hard. People all over the world seem to do it so effortlessly. I had naïvely assumed that parenting would come easy to me. I have always been good with kids, and that's why I initially trained in pediatrics before I did an allergy fellowship. Because I've always had a way with children, I didn't prepare myself for how hard becoming a mother would be.

Parenting is a constant work in progress—an evolution. Parents have to adapt and adjust to our children's ever changing needs. Not having any close relatives with twins I didn't really have anyone to look to for advice, and often these tidbits of advice can make a world of difference. That's why Heather Karpinsky, Jennifer Bright Reach, the Mommy MD Guides team, and I wanted to create something to offer you some pearls of wisdom.

As you read this book keep in mind that every person is different. Your experience is unique. Things may not always progress the way you had planned or expected. You might experience some plateaus and even some setbacks. But know this: You have plenty of company. The best piece of advice I can offer is cut yourself some slack. As mothers, we are constantly worried or feeling guilty about one thing or another. But I truly believe that if children know that they are well loved, everything else is just icing on the cake. You may not always enjoy each and every moment, but they are all worth it!

—Sonal R. Patel, MD

Congratulations on becoming a parent of multiples! This is an exciting time for you and your family. You are starting an amazing journey and this book, *The Mommy MD Guide to Twins, Triplets, and More* will make your first year so much easier.

As a twin mom, I know that the first year is full of love, but it also comes with a lot of challenges. Multiples do not come with an instruction book, although I wish mine did. That is why I wanted to be involved in creating a book that includes everything you need to know about having multiples. Working with these incredible women has been a privilege, and I am so proud of the tips we created to help parents of multiples. You will find help for the *expected* and the *unexpected* as well as ways to keep your multiples safe and healthy, while keeping your sanity.

To create this book, we spoke with 12 Mommy MD Guides—doctors who are also mothers, of multiples. These doctors shared their stories, tips, and tricks about how they made it through parenting multiples.

These smart, funny, fascinating women opened their hearts and lives to us. They shared their challenges and also their celebrations of twins.

The more than 200 tips and stories in this book are presented in the Mommy MD Guides' own words, and each tip is clearly attributed to the doctor who *lived* it. Most of these stories contain kernels of advice. This is what doctors who were expecting did for their own families.

Other stories in this book are just that—true stories. The implied advice is: I made it through this pesky problem, and you can too!

Even though this book is filled with advice from a select group—all Mommy MD Guides—you'll find that they hold vastly differing opinions. We've presented many different viewpoints—but not with the intent to confuse or to offer conflicting advice. Instead, these diverse voices are presented so that you can choose what's best for you as you navigate your own parenting journey.

As you read this book, keep in mind that every person is different. In fact, every *pregnancy* is different. Things change and improve at different speeds for everyone. Not all progress is the same, and not all progress is linear. You might have some ups and downs. You might experience some plateaus—even some setbacks. Know this: You have plenty of company.

Welcome to the Mommy MD Guides!

—Heather Karpinsky

Chapter 1

Pregnancy and Birth

Take all the things a pregnant woman goes through—surprise, excitement, worry, exhaustion, disbelief, shock, joy—and multiply it. Because *you're having multiples!*

The roller coaster of emotions is that much more unpredictable when you're awaiting the arrival of twins, triplets, or quads. Shock might be followed by elation, which may be followed by fear and worry and then more excitement.

Let's start with the surprise. How did this happen? It may have happened two different ways. In one case, one of your eggs was fertilized by sperm and then split into two or three embryos before implanting into the uterine wall. In this case you'll have identical twins or triplets. They will be the same gender and look nearly the same.

Or it may have happened this way. Two or more eggs were released during ovulation, and each was fertilized by different sperm. In this case, you'll have fraternal multiples. They won't look identical and may be the same sex or different sexes.

It's even possible to have multiples in which your

babies are a mix of fraternal and identical. If your body released multiple eggs that were fertilized and one of the eggs divided into two or more embryos, you'll have identical and fraternal multiples.

A multiple pregnancy has its challenges. What may hit first is the fatigue. Women who are pregnant with multiples report extreme sleepiness and exhaustion during the first trimester because the body has to nourish two or more growing babies. Nausea can also be more intense due to higher levels of the pregnancy hormone. And near the end of your pregnancy, you're likely to feel pretty uncomfortable as the babies get bigger—more so than if you were carrying only one.

You might have some worries that you wouldn't necessarily have if you were pregnant with a single baby. Because you're pregnant with multiples, you're at greater risk of having high blood pressure and your babies have a higher risk of being born early and having a low birth weight of 5.5 pounds or less. More than half of twins are born before 37 weeks gestation, and more than 90 percent of triplets, quadruplets, and quintuplets are premature and have low birth weights.

Don't let worry get the best of you. What's most important is keeping yourself healthy during your pregnancy. Be sure to eat nutritious foods, rest, and keep up with your prenatal appointments. Your doctor will tell you how much more to eat to nourish your babies—usually about 300 extra calories a day.

When it's finally time to meet your little one, you might automatically assume you'll be having a Cesarean section, but that's not necessarily the case. When it comes to twins, vaginal delivery is recommended as long as you've reached 32 weeks, the baby closest to the cervix (Baby A) is the largest and is positioned with the head down, and the babies aren't in distress.

〰️

I did IVF, so I found out from the doctor's office that I was having twins. I was over the moon!

—*Jennifer Gilbert, DO, a mom of nine-year-old boy-girl twins and an ob-gyn at Paoli Hospital, in Pennsylvania*

〰️

When I went for my ultrasound, I was able to see two babies before the technician said anything. It felt like an out-of-body experience, as if I were looking at someone else's uterus. I was speechless. The technician also mentioned that they are twin boys (I already had one boy). I just nodded and literally didn't say anything. After a while, I called my husband, and he was over the moon.

—*Saira Butt, MD, a mom of a six-year-old son and three-year-old boy twins and an infectious diseases physician, in Carmel, IN*

Fast Facts

Twins have been shown to begin interacting in the womb as early as 14 weeks.

I have an identical twin sister. I had heard many stories from my mother of how challenging twins are.

When I found out that I was having twins during an early ultrasound, I started to laugh. My husband was in disbelief.

I called my parents and sisters right away to share the news. No one answered the phone. When they called back and I told them, they were all happy—except my mom. Her reaction was, "Oh." I sensed this was not a great thing to her.

The thought that we were going to have twins made me nervous. It wasn't what I had expected. I was very over-whelmed at the thought of having twins. I had to go back to work right after the ultrasound. I was a resident physician, and I had three newly admitted patients waiting for me at the hospital.

Pretty soon, I became comfortable with the idea of having twins. From that point forward, my husband and I were excited about it.

—*Amy J. Lynch, DO, a mom of eight-year-old twin boys and a five-year-old son and a physical medicine and rehabilitation specialist at the Iowa Clinic, in Des Moines*

Fast Facts

If you are a fraternal twin, you have a 1 in 17 chance of having twins.

Fast Facts

The average birth weight for a singleton is 7 pounds 7 ounces. For a twin it's 5 pounds 5 ounces, for triplets 4 pounds, and for quads 3 pounds.

DR. SONAL'S TIPS

When I found out that I was having twins, I was surprised. Two of my cousins have twins, but no one else in the family does.

During the ultrasound, when my doctor told me I was having twins, I asked, "Are you sure?" even though I could clearly see for myself on the monitor. It was hilarious.

As my pregnancy went along, I felt very happy and blessed to be having twins. As an older first-time mother, I knew it was unlikely that there would be other children. I felt grateful to be having two babies in one pregnancy.

I was scared too. I knew that twins are often born prematurely, so I was worried about their health. My age (over 35) automatically put my pregnancy in the high-risk category, and having twins did so even more.

⁓

My husband and I decided to find out the gender of our babies before they were born. We found out ahead of time that both are boys. I'm a planner, and I didn't want any more suspense. I felt that we'd already had our big surprise—learning we were having twins.

—*Amy J. Lynch, DO*

DR. SONAL'S TIPS

My husband and I decided to find out our babies' genders. We wanted to know ahead of time so we could prepare better. One of the biggest requirements for being a twins' parent is being organized.

Because my pregnancy was high risk, I had a CVS (chorionic villus sampling). That's when we found out our babies are girls. Knowing this helped my husband and me to choose names, clothing, and nursery colors.

Because I was eating for three, not just two, I wanted to make sure I was eating enough calories. I used an app to track my food intake. I wanted to balance eating too much versus not enough. My doctor checked my weight at each appointment, of course, and I also kept a chart at home.

Preparing for Baby Safety Checklist

- Take an infant CPR and first aid class before your twins are born—and then commit to retaking it each year.
- Post emergency numbers by each phone: 911, pediatrician, poison control at 800-222-1222, your cell, your partner's cell, and neighbors' cells.
- Enter the emergency numbers into your cell and encourage your partner to do the same.
- Know the route to the closest urgent care and emergency department.
- Install fire alarms on each floor and outside each bedroom.

- Replace the fire alarm batteries yearly; a good time to do this is when you turn your clocks back in the fall.
- Get carbon monoxide alarms.
- Make a fire safety plan.
- Place fire extinguishers in the kitchen, garage, and workshop.
- Practice monthly fire drills.
- Look for the Juvenile Products Manufacturers Association (JPMA) seal on all baby products and gear.
- If you encounter a defect or safety problem with a product, report it to the Consumer Product Safety Commission at CPSC.gov or 800-638-2772.
- Beware of products made before 1973 because federal safety standards didn't take effect until then.
- Make it a habit to check often for product recalls, and sign up for alerts.
- Send in warranty cards for all baby gear that you buy.
- Store batteries far out of reach, especially small ones.
- Get in the habit of keeping balloons and similar plastics far away from children.

Fast Facts

Women who consume a lot of dairy products are five times more likely to have fraternal twins than those who do not.

- *Keep your house clutter-free to prevent falls.*
- *Fasten down rugs.*
- *Clean up spills promptly.*
- *Check your water and paint for lead.*
- *Always tie up plastic grocery bags and store them out of reach of children.*
- *Encourage family and friends to remove their shoes at the door.*
- *Remove rubber knobs from doorstops.*
- *Install baby gates to keep your baby safe from stairs and out of rooms you haven't babyproofed.*
- *Make sure you have a way to unlock all doors in your home in case your baby locks herself in a room.*
- *Keep your home gun- and ammunition-free.*
- *Make your house a smoke-free home.*
- *Create a first aid kit for your home and another for your car, stocked with:*
  - Acetaminophen
  - Adhesive tape
  - Antibiotic ointment
  - Antiseptic cream
  - Band-Aids
  - Cotton
  - Cotton swabs
  - Disposable gloves
  - Dosage spoon for medications
  - Flashlight with working batteries
  - Hydrocortisone cream
  - Scissors with blunt ends
  - Sterile gauze
  - Surgical tape
  - Thermometer
  - Tissues
  - Tweezers

Fast Facts

Extreme fatigue is the most commonly reported complaint during pregnancy with multiples. Sleepiness, lethargy, and exhaustion during the first trimester can be enhanced because the body is working overtime to nurture more than one baby.

DR. SONAL'S TIPS

During my pregnancy, each month or so, my husband and I traced the outline of my belly on the wall, and he'd label it with the date. It was a fun way to monitor my progress. It's still on the wall. My girls love seeing it now.

∽

My best advice to moms-to-be of twins is: It's not going to be perfect. You are going to screw up. I keep a coin jar on my kitchen counter. I tell my kids, "This is for your first therapy session." I'll pay for it; we're going.

> —*Brooke A. Jackson, MD, a mom of 11-year-old twin girls and a 9-year-old son, a dermatologist, and the founder and medical director of the Skin Wellness Dermatology Associates, in Durham, NC*

Dr. Sonal's Tips

One thing that was challenging during my pregnancy was that people always had something to say or some piece of advice to give. I learned to let some of this go in one ear and out the other.

Many times I was told, "Wow, you look so big. You look like you're ready to pop!" When you're nowhere near time to give birth and worried about preterm delivery, that's not exactly something you want to hear.

When I told people I was having twins, they sometimes asked, "Are you sure there aren't three in there?" This was really not funny to me.

It was surprising how often I was asked (even by total strangers), "Did you have IVF?" I felt that it was my choice to decide what information I wanted to disclose.

I tried my best to ignore all of these people.

On the other hand, however, I think it's great to consider family members' opinions and experience. This is valuable. But always remember that you're allowed to make your own choices and do things differently than they did. I remember I once said something to my mother, and she responded back, "I've also raised two daughters. I know what I'm doing." Yes, she did raise two daughters beautifully, in a foreign country without any family support. I respect and appreciate that, but at the same time, I'd like to do things my way.

HEATHER'S TIPS

My twin boys (Grant & Gavin) were born two warriors, arriving at just 31 weeks. My birth story was not the one I had imagined. I think most parents of premature babies feel a little alone and struggle with a lot of different emotions when dealing with a different arrival for their babies than expected. I know I did. It was so hard to see my boys and not be able to hold them. It broke my heart. I instantly loved them with all my heart, but I also felt scared and guilty. I wished during those first couple of days that I had someone to talk to who understood my feelings.

If your twins are in the NICU, ask the nurses if they can organize a meet-up for all the parents, or join an online support group. Making friends with other mothers who had their babies in the NICU really helped me keep my head up during that time. Also, before your twins graduate and leave the NICU, ask the NICU nurses for their email addresses. I can't tell you how many times I emailed our NICU nurse during the first three months at home. Advice is a great thing to have, and having an expert who also knows your children is priceless.

Fast Facts

The location of the baby in the womb denotes which baby is Baby A and which is Baby B. Baby A refers to the baby located lower in the womb, and Baby B refers to the baby who is higher.

Twin to Twin Transfusion Syndrome

Twin to Twin Transfusion Syndrome (TTTS) is a prenatal condition in which twins share unequal amounts of the placenta's blood supply, resulting in the two fetuses growing at different rates. Seventy percent of identical twins share a placenta, and 15 to 20 percent of these pregnancies are affected by TTTS. The condition is not related to anything the mother did or did not do during pregnancy.

If your multiples are being affected by TTTS, you have resources to turn to. The Twin to Twin Transfusion Syndrome Foundation provides educational materials and emotional and financial support. Learn more at **TTTSFOUNDATION.ORG/INDEX.PHP**. The Fetal Health Foundation also provides information on its website and through a newsletter and has a list of treatment centers with a search tab to help you find one near you. For more information, go to **FETALHEALTHFOUNDATION.ORG/FETAL-SYNDROMES/TWIN-TO-TWIN-TRANSFUSION-SYNDROME/**.

Our twins were born a month early. They had problems with temperature regulation and were in the NICU. They needed to be woken up to feed on a schedule for a little while after they came home.

Though it's hard to have your babies in the NICU, it can really be a blessing in disguise. You get time to heal, you have someone to help, and you have time to get them on a schedule. Yes, it's difficult, but for us it was a short time. I was lucky.

Though you will have ups and downs, you'll get through it, one day at a time. Remember, even when your babies are in the NICU, you're still parenting, and you have people to help you. Use them!

—*Cassie Cole, MD, a mom of five-year-old twin girls and an emergency physician, in Hot Springs, AR*

?

When to Call Your Doctor: Premature Labor

Being pregnant with multiples puts you at higher risk for premature labor, which is defined as labor that begins before the 37th week of pregnancy. In fact, 60 percent of multiples are premature, according to the American Society for Reproductive Medicine.

Fortunately, your doctor may be able to prevent premature birth if you catch the warning signs early. The only way to know for sure if you're going into premature labor is to have your doctor check your cervix. Call your doctor right away if you experience these symptoms:

- Five or more contractions an hour, in which you feel your belly become hard and then soft again.
- Leaking fluid from your vagina or any change in vaginal discharge.
- Cramps that are constant or come and go and that may occur with diarrhea.
- A low backache that is constant or comes and goes.
- Pressure in your pelvis that feels like your babies are pushing down.

Fast Facts

A study in the journal *Proceedings of the Royal Society B* suggested healthier moms have twins.

Mommy MD Guides-Recommended Product
Twin Z Pillow

Not everything is more challenging with twins and multiples. Many products are designed with moms and dads of twins/ multiples in mind. The Twin Z Pillow provides ideal support for the nursing mother of multiples and her babies. The Twin Z Pillow is a six-in-one pillow that is perfect for breastfeeding, bottlefeeding, and tummy time and is also great back support for mom. Additionally, it can be used as a sleeping pillow during pregnancy.

As seen on ABC's *Shark Tank*, Twin Z Pillow comes in both a waterproof version that does not require a cover and a white shell pillow that includes a removable cuddle cover. The waterproof material has a soft cotton feel, and the cuddle covers are made of a super-soft material. Additional removable covers are available separately and will fit over the waterproof version of the Twin Z Pillow.

You can find Twin Z Pillows for purchase in a variety of colors on both **AMAZON.COM** and direct from the company's website **TWINZPILLOW.COM**.

I had a very uncomplicated pregnancy. I didn't need to be on bed rest at all. When I was 37 weeks and 4 days pregnant, I was admitted to the hospital after my regular ob-gyn appointment for high blood pressure. They found I was bordering on having HELLP syndrome, which is a serious type of preeclampsia. My babies were induced, and they were then delivered the next day by Cesarean section.

Truth be told, after watching women deliver babies vaginally in medical school, I wanted to have a C-section. I had no desire to work that hard to push a baby out. Because both of my babies were positioned head down, my ob-gyn wanted me to try to deliver vaginally. But despite the fact that the Pitocin was set all the way up, I dilated to only eight centimeters. So my ob-gyn came in at 2:40 in the morning to deliver my babies even though she wasn't on call that night. She's my hero.

—*Amy J. Lynch, DO*

Editor's note: The symptoms of preeclampsia, which is more common in twin pregnancies, are blood pressure of 140/90 mmHg or higher; protein in your urine (checked during your prenatal appointments); headaches; sudden nausea and vomiting halfway through your pregnancy; abdominal pain under your ribs on the right side; lower back pain; weight gain of more than two pounds a week; blurry vision or other changes in vision such as flashing lights or auras and light sensitivity; stronger reflexes; anxiety; shortness of breath; and swelling in your feet, face, and hands.

Fast Facts

Identical twins can have different heights and weights. This is because height and weight are controlled by what you eat as well as your DNA. Differences in diet can start earlier than you might imagine. When the twins are growing inside the uterus, there can be differences in how well they connect to the placenta. This can mean one twin starts getting more to eat even before they are born!

Fast Facts

Twin pregnancies are higher risk than singleton pregnancies. However, moms carrying identical twins are at higher risk of complications than those carrying fraternal. Fraternal twins have their own placentas and their own amniotic sacs. Identicals, on the other hand, can share a placenta, an amniotic sac, and a chorionic sac. Any of these situations increase the risk to the pregnancy. When identical twins share a placenta, they are at risk for Twin to Twin Transfusion Syndrome, or TTTS (a potentially fatal condition where one twin receives more blood from the placenta than the other). In rare situations where twins share a chorionic and amniotic sac, they can also tie their umbilical cords together, risking both of their lives.

DR. SONAL'S TIPS

My twins were born at 36 weeks. I needed to have a C-section, and the recovery from that was harder than expected.

When my twins were born, I had them room in with me. I remember thinking, This is great! *In hindsight, I wish I had sent them to the nursery for a while so I could get some rest. It wouldn't have negatively impacted their bonding time at all.*

After a few days, my girls came home with me from the hospital. Sometimes you have a great plan, but you still may need a backup plan. For the first few weeks after our twins were born,

*my mom stayed with us to help. But when our girls were one
month old, my dad went into acute renal failure. He was hospitalized for three weeks and on dialysis, so my mom had to leave us to
help him. My husband and I were solo for a few weeks, and then
my mother-in-law came to stay with us for a while.*

*Looking back, I wish I would have hired a helper for those
first few months. An overnight nanny would have been ideal so
my husband and I could have gotten some much-needed sleep. I
also felt guilty for not being able to help my dad. We really
struggled those first few months.*

⟳

When my babies were born, my inclination was to keep them in
the room with me. One of my co-residents, who was a new parent too, had strongly recommended sending the twins to the
nursery. "You'll have plenty of time at home with them," she
said. "Get as much sleep as you can in the hospital. Let someone
else take care of your babies while you have the help."

That turned out to be very wise advice.

—*Amy J. Lynch, DO*

Fast Facts

Triplets are far less common than twins. The U.S.
Centers for Disease Control and Prevention reports
that 1 in 1,000 births is triplets. Of these births, 10
percent are identical triplets.

When it came time to choose our babies' names, my husband and I simply picked two names we liked the best. I'm a child of the '80s, and my twin and I are Angela and Amy. I made a point to avoid naming my kids with rhyming or same-first-letter names.

—*Amy J. Lynch, DO*

Get a Prenatal Spa Treatment

Life is about to change in a big way—or two, three, or more! These last weeks of your pregnancy are the perfect time for some pampering before the really hard work begins—and salons and spas have you covered with plenty of prenatal services.

Studies have found prenatal massage to be beneficial to your health. It relieves anxiety and depression symptoms and eases sore muscles and joints. It may even lead to a better labor and make your newborn healthier!

Choose a relaxing prenatal massage, facial, or body, hand, or foot treatment. And if you're getting a massage, be sure your therapist is certified in prenatal massage. It's also a good idea to check with your doctor first to be sure it's safe for you.

When my twins came home from the hospital, my mother came to stay with us for the first week or two. As a mom of twins herself, she jumped right in to help. She wasn't overwhelmed by caring for two babies at once. I had complete confidence in her, and she was an excellent help.

—*Amy J. Lynch, DO*

My children are adopted. I didn't take maternity leave. We brought the babies home on the weekend, and I was back to work on Thursday.

One of the things I tell newly adoptive moms is don't shortchange yourself. You deserve maternity leave, and you deserve a baby shower.

—*Brooke A. Jackson, MD*

Fast Facts

- If twins are present on your partner's side, it won't influence your chances of having twins. The gene for hyperovulation is only a factor for the mother.

- The odds of having twins born in different years are 1 in 1,984,262.

- A 15-year German study of 8,220 vaginally delivered twins yielded a mean delivery time interval of 13.5 minutes. The delivery interval results are:
  - ★ Within 15 minutes: 75.8 percent
  - ★ 16 to 30 minutes: 16.4 percent
  - ★ 31 to 45 minutes: 4.3 percent
  - ★ 46 to 60 minutes: 1.7 percent
  - ★ More than 60 minutes: 1.8 percent

- Cassandra Flores gave birth to her twins Israel at 1:39 p.m. and Isaiah at 1:40 p.m. at St. Joseph Hospital in Orange, California, on July 9, 2013. Their birth was natural and is the shortest amount of time between twin births.

- Maria Jones-Elliot gave birth to twins Amy Ann and Kate Marie Elliot 87 days apart, making them the twins with the longest interval between their births. The twins were born at Waterford Regional Hospital in Ireland. Amy was born prematurely on June 1, 2012, and Kate followed on August 27. Because Amy Ann was born at 9:16 and Kate Marie at 11:01, the exact interval is 87 days, 1 hour and 45 minutes.

Fast Facts

- Born September 4, 2004, Rumasia Rahman is currently the world's smallest premature baby to have survived from birth until hospital discharge. Rumasia and her fraternal twin sister Hiba were born at 25.6 weeks gestation. At birth, Rumasia weighed just 8.6 ounces and was 9.8 inches long. Rumasia's twin sister Hiba was more than twice her size, at 1 pound 4 ounces and 12 inches long.
- Mirror image twins are monozygotic, twins that form from a single fertilized egg. When the split occurs late—more than a week after conception—the twins can develop reverse asymmetric features.
- In very rare cases, identical twins can have different hair and eye color. This result is from incongruities in how pigment-forming cells migrate through the body during growth.
- Fraternal twins can have different blood types.
- Identical twins do not have identical fingerprints, even though their identical genes give them very similar patterns. From the early weeks of pregnancy when a fetus is developing fingerprint patterns, small differences in the womb cause each twin to have different (but similar) fingerprints.
- Cryptophasia is a secret language developed by twins (identical or fraternal) that only the two children can understand. The word has its roots from *crypto*, meaning secret, and *phasia*, meaning speech.

Chapter 2

Feeding

Breast milk provides the perfect meal for your babies—protein, sugar, and fat—and delivers substances that help boost your babies' immune systems and help protect them against allergies, diseases, and infection. If your babies were premature, breast milk is also easier on their tummies, which are still maturing, and helps their intestines continue to develop.

That said, it can be difficult to breastfeed premature babies. Babies born before 37 weeks may not be able to suck and swallow or have the reflexes to latch onto the breast. However, it is possible for a baby who is at least 28 weeks gestation to breastfeed, at least briefly.

There are a few things you can do to help breastfeeding go more smoothly when you have premature babies. Even if your babies are whisked away to the NICU right after birth, expressing milk within an hour of giving birth will produce creamy colostrum that can be given to your babies with a syringe. Having skin-to-skin contact as often as possible may also help, including when your babies are getting treatment through intravenous fluids or ventilation. Ask the nurse how your babies should be positioned so their necks and airways are supported. If your babies are receiving tube feeding, they can practice breastfeeding at the same time by sucking on the breast or your finger.

You might also wonder if you can produce enough milk for multiples. The answer is yes! The more you breast-feed, the more milk you'll produce. To get your milk flowing, start breastfeeding or pumping with a hospital-grade breast pump soon after your babies are born and do it 8 to 12 times each 24-hour period.

If your babies are ready to breastfeed, start by feeding them one at a time so you can watch how they latch on. It's a good idea to track how long each baby nurses on a chart, along with how many wet and dirty diapers they have. (See Chapter 3 for where to find a chart to print out or which apps can help you do this.)

Once your babies have learned to latch on and are breastfeeding well, it's okay to feed two at a time if you prefer. You can do this with the double football hold, using a pillow for each baby to lie on under each arm. Or you can cradle one baby and have the other in a football hold. Another option is the double-cradle hold, in which both babies are cradled in front of you with their legs on top of each other creating an "X."

If breastfeeding your multiples is a struggle, meet with

a lactation consultant who has experience with multiples for help. Remember, there's no shame in using formula or using a combination of breast milk and formula if that's what's needed to help your babies grow.

～

I placed my twins side by side to feed. I fed them by holding a bottle in each of my hands at the same time.

—*Saira Butt, MD, a mom of three-year-old twins and an infectious diseases physician, in Carmel, IN*

～

When my twins were babies, I would set up a feeding station before I went to bed. I got their bottles ready and set out their clean diapers and clothes for changing. I could do an entire feeding, burping, and changing in 10 minutes. Being organized really helps.

—*Jennifer Gilbert, DO, a mom of nine-year-old boy-girl twins and an ob-gyn at Paoli Hospital, in Pennsylvania*

～

We put our twins on the same schedule. When one twin woke to eat, the other twin was fed too.

I have an incredibly involved husband and took advantage of his willingness to take turns with feeds. We also allowed other family members to help with feeding them. At first that was pumped breast milk, and then later formula.

—*Anne Rodrigue, DO, a mom of two-year-old twin girls and an ob-gyn at Thibodaux Women's Center, in Louisiana*

I set the expectation early on that my husband and I were equal partners in caring for our twins. I knew that I wasn't going to be able to do this by myself. I let him know he was expected to help me in the middle of the night.

We both were working full-time, but I was on maternity leave. He worked from home, traveling occasionally. When he was home, he helped me feed the boys during the day, which was a huge help.

—*Amy J. Lynch, DO, a mom of eight-year-old twin boys and a five-year-old son and a physical medicine and rehabilitation specialist at the Iowa Clinic, in Des Moines*

When my twins were babies, I had a feeding schedule in the kitchen. I measured the formula before going to bed, so at night we only had to add water and shake it up.

It was tricky to keep track of how much formula each girl drank. I kept a chart in the kitchen. (I was type A, so why not?) I would think that I had fed one baby and would wonder why she was still hungry. *Oh, crap,* I'd think, *I fed her sister twice.* You really can't rely on your brain at this time in your life. You have to rely on pen and paper.

I also kept a book in my kitchen I called "the twin book." It was filled with notes to babysitters about what they liked to eat, what soothed them, etc.

—*Brooke A. Jackson, MD, a mom of 11-year-old twin girls and a 9-year-old son, a dermatologist, and the founder and medical director of the Skin Wellness Dermatology Associates, in Durham, NC*

For bottle feedings, I used the Twin Z pillow (*TwinZNursingPillow .com*), and I held the bottles. (See the Mommy MD Guides— Recommended Product box on page 31.)

> —*Leah Cobb, MD, a mom of 20-month-old twins and a pediatric orthopedic surgeon at San Jorge Children's Hospital, in San Juan, PR*

The Twin Z pillow was and still is our lifesaver. It is adjustable and grows with the boys. The boys have had most of their bottles in that pillow, and I was also able to use it for breastfeeding.

> —*Andrea Orr, MD, a mom of 10-month-old twin boys and a pediatrician with Northwest Pediatrics Washington University Clinical Associates, in St. Louis, MO*

With twins you need two feeding pillows. We had two Boppys. I'd "wear" one Boppy around me and put the other on the floor. This way, I could feed one twin while the other was resting comfortably on the other pillow.

> —*Brooke A. Jackson, MD*

I found the Twin Z pillow was a big help at feeding time, as we would position it on the couch and be able to feed both babies simultaneously. After they had a little more head control, I was even able to pump at the same time. It became such a big part of feedings that the girls continued to use it to drink their bottles, then their milk in cups, until just recently.

> —*Anne Rodrigue, DO*

As a mom of twins, you learn how to use all of your limbs. We had a baby rocker that moved from side to side. I'd hold one, put the other in the rocker, and rock it with my foot.

—*Brooke A. Jackson, MD*

A lot of people advise moms of twins to feed them both at the same time. I found it more helpful to stagger them by 15 to 20 minutes—especially if I was home alone with them. I'd feed one, burp her, and then put her down and take a little break before it was time to do it all for the second twin.

—*Brooke A. Jackson, MD*

My twins were NICU babies, and they didn't latch well. I never had the energy to do a billion lactation appointments. When my twins were infants, I pumped exclusively.

—*Leah Cobb, MD*

Talk to someone who has successfully breastfed. (I had my older sister.) Avoid talking with people who have not done it and will discourage you.

—*Maria Peters, MD, a mom of five-year-old boy/girl twins and an ophthalmologist in private practice in Los Angeles, CA*

Mommy Time: Go for a Run

When we adopted our girls, I was training for a marathon. My running group ran each Saturday morning, and that was my time.

—Brooke A. Jackson, MD

Fast Facts

Numerous studies have been done on fraternal and identical twins to see if they have the same allergies. Fraternal twins are far less likely to share the same allergies (for example, same peanut allergy, 7 percent) than identical twins (same peanut allergy, 65 percent). Also, identical twins may be sensitive to the same allergens, but their symptoms may differ. For instance, one may get a mild skin rash, while the other may suffer from respiratory distress.

My twins were born prematurely. We had lots of problems breast-feeding, particularly with their latch and my milk supply. I really wanted to breastfeed them together at the same time, but as soon as I got the second baby latched on, the first would pop off.

Because we were supplementing with bottles, I eventually realized that I could tandem feed them differently: I breastfed one twin while I bottlefed the other, then I'd switch.

With twins it's important to be creative and think outside the box. I used my legs for things I never would have thought of otherwise, including holding the baby who was getting the bottle while the other one was breastfeeding. I also sometimes held my babies with my legs while I was pumping because my hands were occupied.

—Valerie Sheppard, MD, a mom of five-year-old boy/girl twins and a pediatrician with Newport Children's Medical Group, in Newport Beach, CA

I struggled a lot to establish nursing with my first daughter. Looking back, I can see that I set myself up for failure by assuming it would be easy.

In fact, feeding was the hardest part of those first few months! It affected everything I did. I didn't want to leave the house for fear that the baby wouldn't eat enough. I didn't want to give her formula because I had convinced myself that using formula meant I had failed.

I obsessed over my daughter's weight gain. It consumed me.

I learned a lot from that experience. Although over time we were very successful, I never wanted to repeat that tension and worry. I was so stressed, and I know my baby could sense it.

Mommy MD Guides–Recommended Product
The Twin Feeding Set from BabyA-BabyB.com

The Twin Feeding Set is the only feeding system invented for the needs of twins. It solves the problem all twin parents face: how to feed two babies at once. Creator and mother of twins—and this book's coauthor—Heather Karpinsky designed this product to protect her twin boys. It makes feeding time easier, safer, and faster. The Twin Feeding Set can be purchased online at **BABYA-BABYB.COM** and **WALMART.COM**.

When I got pregnant the second time and discovered we were having twins, I didn't set any expectations for nursing. I planned to pump from the get-go and supplement when we needed it, which we did. My boy twin ended up in the NICU for a week and a half. During that time, both twins received some formula and some breast milk that I had been able to pump.

Pumping right away helped me establish a good supply and ensured that my babies were getting enough—so I didn't worry. When my twins were around five weeks old, we were able to establish exclusive nursing.

We worked very closely with a lactation consultant. She helped me with my first baby, and I made sure that she was available to help me with the twins. The best advice I have for a mom who wants to nurse twins? Take every day as it comes, and never quit on a bad day.

—*Meredith Brauer, MD, a mom of a three-year-old daughter and six-month-old boy-girl twins and an internal medicine hospitalist at Central DuPage Hospital, in Winfield, IL*

❧

My twins were born at 36 weeks. They didn't learn to breastfeed until they were six weeks old. We did "triple feeds" where I had them practice at the breast, then I'd use a hands-free pump, prop them in the Twin Z pillow, and give them the milk from the last pumping session at the same time I pumped.

Thank goodness they finally learned to latch and take milk from the breast. We used the Twin Z and My Brest Friend twin nursing pillows for almost a year until they outgrew them. When they started eating solids, we quickly moved from mushed-up food to baby-led weaning. Feeding two babies and myself at meal time? Ain't nobody got time for that!

—Megan Lemay, MD, a mom of a three-year-old son and 22-month-old twin boys and an assistant professor of internal medicine at the Virginia Commonwealth University School of Medicine, in Richmond

I was a resident when my twins were born, and I breastfed. We used a Boppy pillow with pillows around and on the bed. If one twin woke early, I fed that twin, then the other one. I had to do triple feeds in the beginning, and I pumped for when I was away at work. It does get easier. Remember that breastfeeding is wonderful, but fed babies and mother's mental health are the most important priorities. After all, you need a happy, healthy mom for happy, healthy babies.

—Cassie Cole, MD, a mom of five-year-old twins and an emergency physician, in Hot Springs, AR

My boys were both breast- and formula-fed until they were seven and a half months old. Now they're exclusively on formula. We use a Dr. Brown's formula mixing pitcher to make several bottles at a time.

—*Andrea Orr, MD*

I fed my twins formula from the beginning. The thought of breastfeeding two babies was completely overwhelming to me.

Formula-fed babies can go longer between feedings than breastfed babies, so my babies were able to make it four hours between feedings pretty early on. I got them onto a feeding schedule of 6 a.m., 10 a.m., 2 p.m., 6 p.m., 10 p.m., 2 a.m. by around three to four weeks—very quickly.

I would stay up until 10 p.m. to feed them, then wake up at 2 a.m. to feed. By 6 a.m. it was time to get up anyway. We were lucky to have good sleepers.

—*Amy J. Lynch, DO*

MomMy TIME Celebrate Breaking Up with Your Breast Pump

Frankly, I didn't make much time for myself until I stopped pumping when my twins were 12 months old. It's amazing how freeing it is to be done pumping and to have three or four hours of time back each day! That's definitely worth a celebration!

The few times I did make time for myself in the first year, I asked our nanny to stay late on my afternoon off, and instead of rushing home to take care of my twins, I did something fun for myself.

—Valerie Sheppard, MD

Dr. Sonal's Tips

I really wanted to breastfeed, but it was very challenging for me. Now I wish I had seen a lactation specialist. Many insurance companies cover visits, and your pediatrician can probably refer you to one. I blame myself for not asking for help because I thought breastfeeding would come naturally.

I could have used a lactation specialist's expert advice and tips. People think doctors know these things, but we aren't trained in breastfeeding. I was so tired, in a brain fog, and struggling that it didn't occur to me to see a specialist.

Instead, I stressed myself greatly trying to breastfeed when I wasn't producing enough milk for both girls. This is a common challenge for moms of twins—the need to produce more milk. Of course, the stress didn't help my milk production any. I obsessed over the girls' lack of weight gain.

I tried many things to increase my breast milk supply, including taking the herbs milk thistle and fenugreek, but nothing seemed to work. I felt so guilty for not being able to breastfeed more. I was also resistant to formula feeding.

For a little while, we kept a chart to track which baby had fed, for how long, and from which breast. I discovered that one breast was producing more milk than the other.

Both twins were gaining weight slowly, so the doctor needed to monitor their weight carefully. She gave me "permission" to supplement with formula. My girls had been given some formula already in the hospital because one of them had jaundice, so the nurses needed to encourage her to eat and to poop. I introduced formula to my twins fairly early. Sometimes I think my mom gave them formula in the night because she felt so bad waking me up. She was using her mom instincts, knowing I needed my rest. Plus, I had been a formula-fed baby. (And I turned out all right!) Back then, formula feeding was de rigueur. For a while I did a combo of feeding breast milk and formula. I fed each baby on one breast and then finished each with a bottle. We had a Twin Z Pillow and two Boppys, which were kindly donated to me by other mommies.

This quickly presented a challenge! Because I had planned to breastfeed, I didn't have any bottles—other than the two-ounce ones they had given us at the hospital. For a person like me who likes to be prepared, I was quite unprepared! I experimented with a few brands of bottles until I found one bottle my girls liked. Then I bought about a dozen of them, plenty for both babies for an entire day. This way I didn't have to stress about cleaning them up all of the time.

Fast Facts

A study looked at the mouth bacteria of 485 sets of twins (205 sets of identical twins and 280 nonidentical twins) in Australia and found that some mouth bacteria is inherited, but not the ones that cause tooth decay. Bacteria starts growing even before the teeth appear, and diet, even when they are toothless, can influence children's future oral health. When teeth do emerge, their condition depends upon diet and oral hygiene.

When to Call Your Doctor: Illness

Don't play a guessing game if you're worried one of your babies could be sick. Call your pediatrician if your baby is less than three months old and has a temperature of 100.4°F or higher; your baby is three to six months old and has a fever over 102°F or has a lower fever and seems sick; your baby is six to 24 months old and has a fever higher than 102°F that lasts longer than a day, even if there are no other symptoms of illness; or if any fever lasts more than three days.

Other signs of illness that warrant a call to the doctor include poor appetite; crying more than usual and difficulty calming down; extreme sleepiness and having trouble waking; an oozing or red area around the umbilical cord or penis; diarrhea or vomiting (not spit up), especially if your baby hasn't kept liquids down for eight hours; fewer than your baby's usual number of bowel movements for a few days; fewer wet diapers; a dry mouth; crying without tears; trouble

So I could tell which bottle was whose, I color-coded them. One girl used bottles with a pink cap; the other used blue.

As I used formula, I discovered that it was quick to premeasure a bunch of powder into the clean bottles. Then when I needed to make a bottle, I just had to add the water. It's great when taking the babies out also.

I used a hands-free pumping bra while I was at work.

breathing because of a cold; nasal mucus for more than 10 days; a cough that lasts longer than a week; ear pain (indicated such as by tugging on her ear); a sudden rash or a rash that looks infected; or eyes that look red or have discharge.

Call 911 if your child experiences any of the following:

- A seizure
- Extreme trouble breathing
- Bleeding that won't stop
- Accidental poisoning
- Vomiting after a head injury
- Deep cuts or burns
- Smoke inhalation
- Blue, purple, or gray lips or skin
- Near drowning
- Severe pain or injuries to the mouth or face
- Unconsciousness

I chugged along trying to continue pumping and giving breast milk too until the girls were about 10 months old, but then I had to stop breastfeeding. I wasn't producing any milk, and it wasn't worth all the time I was spending pumping and washing the pump. I had been back to work for a few months, and it was hard. I was driving myself mad to produce very little milk. When I stopped breastfeeding my twins, I felt a mixture of sadness and relief.

I relied on two bottle warmers that could be used simulta-neously. This was especially helpful when I was warming thawed/stored breast milk and during nighttime feeds.

—*Anne Rodrigue, DO*

∽

I started solids when my twins were four months old. I made homemade foods with a Baby Brezza (BabyBrezza.com). This is a handy, easy-to-use appliance that cooks food and blends it in one step.

Today, my twins eat everything—except chicken nuggets and mac and cheese! But I still haven't figured out how to get them to sit at the table and eat.

—*Leah Cobb, MD*

MomMy TIME **Load Up Your Netflix Queue**

You're likely spending lots of time rocking, feeding, burping, and just chilling with a little one (or two) asleep on your shoulder. When you're not gazing into your babies' beautiful eyes, you could take this opportunity to catch up on some uplifting movies on your favorite streaming service or from a DVD rental box.

If you're looking for a movie with a twin theme, try these films:

- *Twinsters*
- *The Parent Trap*
- *It Takes Two*
- *Twins*
- *Twin Sisters*
- *Double Identity: The Mystery of Twins*

For other inspiring films, old and new, consider these:

- *Hidden Figures*
- *Mamma Mia!*
- *Julie & Julia*
- *Life of Pi*
- *The Pursuit of Happyness*
- *Beaches*
- *A Room with a View*
- *Dreamgirls*
- *Titanic*
- *The Color Purple*
- *The Bridges of Madison County*
- *Love Actually*
- *When Harry Met Sally*
- *Ghost*
- *Big Fish*
- *Les Misérables*
- *Breakfast at Tiffany's*
- *Coco before Chanel*
- *Chocolat*
- *Mona Lisa Smile*
- *Dirty Dancing*
- *Girl with a Pearl Earring*

Chapter 3

Diapering and Dressing

Get ready for diaper changes. One newborn baby needs about 10 diaper changes a day, so if you just gave birth to twins, you'll be changing upward of 20 or more diapers in 24 hours. If you have triplets, you'll be wiping bottoms and grabbing new diapers 30 times a day! You'll be a pro by the end of the first day, and by the time your babies are two months old, you'll have changed thousands of diapers. If friends and family ask what you may need as a baby gift when they come to visit, you could suggest a box of diapers, because twins go through 4,800 diapers by their first birthday.

Wet versus dry diapers are also a clue into how well your babies are eating, especially if you're breastfeeding and can't tell how much milk they're drinking. During the first couple of days, your babies will have only one or two wet diapers each day. But on the third day, that number will go up to about six a day. They also should have their first bowel movement within the first eight hours, followed by about three bowel movements a day during the first week.

It's a good idea to keep track of how long your babies are nursing or how many ounces they drink from a bottle, along with how many wet or soiled diapers they have in a day. You could designate a notebook to store this information or print out a daily feeding and diapering chart. There are loads of online charts you can print. You can also find feeding and diapering charts in this document from the U.S. Department of Health and Human Services Office on Women's Health: uhs.berkeley.edu/sites/default/files/wellness-womenshealth_breastfeedingguide_0.pdf.

Another simple way to track feedings and diapers is through an app. The Eat Sleep Poop app is free and is so simple that using it is no problem when you're sleep deprived. You can create a profile for each baby and simply tap the buttons on the screen to track your babies' feeds, wet and dirty diapers, and medications. Learn more here: http://eat-sleeppoopapp.com. Another free option in the app store is Baby Tracker, which helps you track feedings and diaper changes, has built-in sleep alarms, and has an extra dim night mode. It can be used with more than one baby. To find out more, go here: http://nighp.com/babytracker.

Or you could get high-tech. Hatch Baby offers a smart changing pad that weighs your babies and can be paired with a free app that will help you track diapers, feedings, and growth. The changing pad can be used with a maximum of two babies and costs $129, while the app is free. To learn more, go here: http://app.hatchbaby.com/#firstPage.

We always changed our twins on the floor to make sure nobody fell off the table while we changed the other!

> —*Megan Lemay, MD, a mom of a three-year-old son and 22-month-old twin boys and an assistant professor of internal medicine at the Virginia Commonwealth University School of Medicine, in Richmond*

Before my twins were mobile, I kept one twin in the Twin Z pillow, placed on the floor, while I diapered the other one.

Once my twins were mobile, I put one in a bouncy seat next to me on the floor while I changed the other.

> —*Leah Cobb, MD, a mom of 20-month-old twins and a pediatric orthopedic surgeon at San Jorge Children's Hospital, in San Juan, PR*

We used Pampers Swaddlers diapers. We tried everything else, and they were the only diapers that didn't leak.

> —*Amy J. Lynch, DO, a mom of eight-year-old twin boys and a five-year-old son and a physical medicine and rehabilitation specialist at the Iowa Clinic, in Des Moines*

Be prepared to go through lots and lots of diapers. We used so many diapers, I started saving the boxes and made them into a castle for my twins to play in!

> —*Valerie Sheppard, MD, a mom of five-year-old boy/girl twins and a pediatrician with Newport Children's Medical Group, in Newport Beach, CA*

I kept it simple. I used diaper rash cream only when needed. Otherwise, I gave my babies a quick wipe-down, patted their skin with the new diaper, and then put it on.

—*Saira Butt, MD, a mom of a six-year-old son and three-year-old boy twins and an infectious diseases physician, in Carmel, IN*

 ⁓

DR. SONAL'S TIPS

I was lucky that my babies rarely got diaper rash. I tried to keep on top of diaper changes. I also used Vaseline prophylactically. I admit I didn't have 100 percent compliance. One of my daughters had extremely sensitive skin, and she was prone to rashes.

Sometimes I spread the Vaseline or diaper rash cream on the clean diaper before undressing my baby. Then when I slid the diaper on, it was already ready. I didn't need to fidget with the diaper rash cream tube.

 ⁓

As environmentally unfriendly as it was, we used disposable diapers and a wipe warmer. One of our twins had sensitive skin, so we switched to using unscented wipes, butt creams, and other skin care products for both of them.

—*Anne Rodrigue, DO, a mom of two-year-old twin girls and an ob-gyn at Thibodaux Women's Center, in Louisiana*

My advice? Don't change diapers overnight unless they're poopie. The babies will be fine in a wet diaper. Just slather diaper cream on their bottoms before bed. That way, it's easier to feed them in the middle of the night and put them back down to sleep—and easier for you to sleep as well!

—*Cassie Cole, MD, a mom of five-year-old twin girls and an emergency physician, in Hot Springs, AR*

Make sure you have a diaper disposal receptacle (a Diaper Genie, trash can, etc.) on each floor. You don't want to be carrying two babies up and down stairs for diaper changes!

—*Valerie Sheppard, MD*

We have a changing station on each floor of our house, so that no matter where you are, there's a supply of diapers and wipes within reach. Keep in mind—especially if you're having boy-girl twins—you may need different-size diapers at different times, due to weight differences.

—*Meredith Brauer, MD, a mom of a three-year-old daughter and six-month-old boy-girl twins and an internal medicine hospitalist at Central DuPage Hospital, in Winfield, IL*

I had two diaper changing stations—one in the living room and one in the twins' nursery. The changing station in the living room helped a ton! I kept them stocked with diapers, wipes, and cream.

—*Leah Cobb, MD*

We have a diaper station or area in each of the main places we play or hang out with our twins in the house. However, more often than not, we change them both quickly on the changing table in their room before or after they sleep. It's usually easier for us to use the changing table in their room so that we can place the other child in his crib, especially now that they're mobile.

—*Andrea Orr, MD, a mom of 10-month-old twin boys and a pediatrician with Northwest Pediatrics Washington University Clinical Associates, in St. Louis, MO*

Mommy MD Guides-Recommended Product
Diaper Subscription to the Honest Company

The Honest Company was "built by parents for parents." They provide essential family necessities directly to your door. The company offers a Diapers and Wipes Bundle that allows you to cross one essential thing off your to-do list. You start by signing up for a "trial kit" that allows you to sample some of their products. Then you fill out a profile that helps them determine which products are right for you. With the Diapers and Wipes Bundle, you get six packs of stylish diapers and four packs of soft, plant-based wipes. Depending on size, you get at least 240 diapers per bundle. You can update your preferences and adjust your ship dates at any time, and you always get free refunds and returns. You can cancel at any time. They also offer Organic Formula Bundle Packs as well. The Diapers and Wipes Bundle is $79.95 at **Honest.com**.

DR. SONAL'S TIPS

When I was younger, I was in Greenpeace, so I wish I could say I used cloth diapers. But we didn't. I used disposable diapers and a wipe warmer. I ran out of time checking into other options before my twins were born. I think using cloth diapers is doable—even with twins. But because I hadn't prepared ahead of time, once my babies were born, it was too hard to check into it.

When our twins were babies, we changed their diapers "assembly-line" style. This worked out best when I had someone to help me—my husband or my mom. I would feed one twin and then hand the baby off to my husband or mom to change while I fed the other twin. Then I'd hand that baby off for a diaper change.

With twins, I think it's especially important to have every-thing you need close by for diaper changes. I stocked two diaper changing stations with wipes, diapers, Vaseline, and ointment.

One of the diaper changing stations was in our master bedroom. It's not a good idea to change a diaper in the dark, yet if you turn on the full light, it can wake up everyone in the room. So my husband attached a book light to the changing table. That little light provided just enough light to change the diapers.

I also kept a diaper changing caddy in our living room. This way we didn't always have to go to their bedroom to change them. This was key, especially when one twin was napping in the bedroom.

I changed so many diapers that I got to be very fast! Before undressing the baby, I unfolded the clean diaper and had it ready to go. I even got wipes out of the container. I took off the dirty diaper and cleaned the baby fast. Then I slid the clean diaper on and secured it.

MomMy TIME

Let the Chores Slide Sometimes

Finding time for myself is still a work in progress. Some days the only five minutes I get to myself is in the bathroom! I think this is true for most moms, but obviously it can be more difficult for moms of multiples. Some days I'll ask my husband if I could have an hour to go do something on my own, such as make a run to Target or the grocery store, or get a manicure or pedicure. We hired a nanny for child care, and some days I'm home from work, but we still have her at the house to free me up to accomplish things I can do only by myself.

Also, whenever we make the impossible happen and all three kids are sleeping at the same time, guess what I do? I sleep! I try not to think that every free moment should be filled with cleaning or cooking or shopping for the family. I let some of that go so that I can sit and binge-watch a show or read a book, and that keeps me sane.

—Meredith Brauer, MD

DR. SONAL'S TIPS

When my girls started to potty train, we bought a training potty. I lined it with a diaper. This made cleanup easier.

We just kept our babies in pajamas all day every day, so we never had to get them into new clothes!

—*Megan Lemay, MD*

∽

I made dressing my twins extra easy by not using onesies or button-downs that required extra time. Just pull-on clothes for us!

—*Saira Butt, MD*

∽

For my twins' first few months, if we weren't leaving the house, they stayed in their jammies all day! It's easy to get pajamas zippered up and down, as opposed to worrying about snapping onesies and putting pants back on squirmy babies.

—*Meredith Brauer, MD*

∽

While you're dressing one baby, make sure the other is safe by putting the second baby on a safe surface such as in a crib, in a Pack 'n Play, etc. I did have the conversation with the babies when they were fussing while I was tending to one that there was one mommy and two babies!

—*Cassie Cole, MD*

∽

Our routine is to dress our twins right after their morning nap. This way the child not being dressed stays in his crib until it's his turn. We generally dress them in the same or a coordinating outfit. That's the fun part about having twins!

—*Andrea Orr, MD*

I'm a twin myself, and my mom sometimes dressed my sister and me alike. It didn't cause any resentment on my part, so I dressed my boys alike early on. It helped me to monitor what was dirty and when I had to do the laundry.

—*Amy J. Lynch, DO*

DR. SONAL'S TIPS

A big question with twins is whether or not to dress them alike. I do a mix of both. I remember when my girls were about three years old, a fellow twin mother commented to me, "I can't tell your girls apart because you dress them alike." I was a little surprised to hear that from another twin mother. Siblings who are not twins often dress alike.

Now that my girls are older, sometimes they like to dress alike. And dressing them alike does make for cute photos.

But dressing them differently helps people to tell them apart. It helps them develop their own identity. Plus, you can't always have two of everything!

Our twins mommy group does a biannual clothing exchange. This was a great way to get clothing in great condition and donate items my babies had outgrown.

Fast Facts

The average number of diapers needed for the first year for twins is 4,800!

Fast Facts

Newborns (one to two months old) average about 10 diaper changes a day per baby. That equals around 20 changes a day for twins. That means at two months old, twins will have used around 1,200 diapers.

I gave up on having my twins wear matching outfits very quickly. They generally would start the day matching, but if one had an accident, I let them be different.

I made an exception for big events, such as holidays, larger family gatherings, and family photos. The key was always having two of each outfit so if one got messed up, I could change both of them.

—*Anne Rodrigue, DO*

∽

My husband and I dressed our twins alike at first until they were older and had opinions. After that, anything goes.

—*Cassie Cole, MD*

∽

I never dressed my twins the same. I don't think that's fair. They're two separate people.

—*Brooke A. Jackson, MD, a mom of 11-year-old twin girls and a 9-year-old son, a dermatologist, and the founder and medical director of the Skin Wellness Dermatology Associates, in Durham, NC*

When your twins are a bit older and stop going through spare outfits so often when you take them out, save space in your diaper bag by having just one extra outfit that either of them could wear. I also keep a spare set of clothes for each of my kids in my car just in case, though.

—*Valerie Sheppard, MD, a mom of five-year-old boy/girl twins and a pediatrician with Newport Children's Medical Group, in Newport Beach, CA*

When my boys were babies, all of their clothing was shared. I kept it all in the same dresser.

Now my boys have their own rooms, and they no longer share clothing. I can't keep their clothing straight anymore, so I keep their laundry separate. Even this morning, my one son brought a shirt to me and said, "You mixed up our shirts." Each boy has a laundry basket in his room, and I do their laundry separately.

I just do each boy's clothing in one load on "regular" wash. They grow out of it so quickly, I'm not worried about it getting ruined in the wash.

—*Amy J. Lynch, DO*

Fast Facts

It takes approximately two to five minutes to change a diaper. That means parents of twins spend 160 hours to 400 hours a year changing diapers.

Clothes shopping with boy-girl twins is challenging. My first strategy is to shop at stores that sell both boy and girl kids' clothing, like Gymboree. My second strategy is to buy in bulk.

Each season I go through their closets, pull out what doesn't fit, donate it, and replace it with new clothing. Now that my kids are older, I buy a lot of their clothing online. This works well if you're very familiar with a brand, such as the Under Armour brand that my son wears frequently.

—*Jennifer Gilbert, DO, a mom of nine-year-old boy-girl twins and an ob-gyn at Paoli Hospital, in Pennsylvania*

With twins, you go through a lot of clothing. My boys basically wear the same size.

To save money, I sign up for e-mails at kids' clothing stores. When I get sales e-mails, I stock up on jeans and other essentials. I buy a season ahead, so in spring I buy winter coats, one size larger than what they're currently wearing.

—*Amy J. Lynch, DO*

I used a lot of hand-me-down clothes from moms in the twins club I joined. Your precious babies look cute in anything!

—*Maria Peters, MD, a mom of five-year-old boy/girl twins and an ophthalmologist in private practice in Los Angeles, CA*

MomMy TIME **Delegate**

Include your partner and ask for specific help. You don't have to parent alone, and it is easier for everyone if there is no guessing involved.

When you're exhausted and stressed, it's easy for miscommunications to happen. For example, my husband thought that I wanted to be the only one to bathe our twins, which couldn't have been farther from the truth. I didn't enjoy bath time, but he loved it. As soon as we realized this, my husband became the primary person to bathe our babies, which was a big help to me.

—Valerie Sheppard, MD, a mom of five-year-old boy/ girl twins and a pediatrician with Newport Children's Medical Group in Newport Beach, CA

Chapter 4

Sleeping

One thing on every new parent's mind is, *how will I get my babies to sleep through the night?* When you have two or more, it makes getting on a sleep schedule all that more complicated. Often one twin will begin sleeping through the night before the other, and you may worry that one crying baby will wake a sibling.

Where you decide to have your multiples sleep can have an impact on your nights. Should they be together in the same bassinet or separate? Your babies were together in the womb and may sleep better when they're close, or your babies may wake each other and will sleep better with some distance. It's a decision you can make based on what's best for you and your babies.

Know that it is okay to have them sleep together in one bassinet until they are around six months old and begin moving around more at night.

For safe co-sleeping, put your babies down on their backs, either side by side or with their heads facing each other and their feet at opposite ends of the bassinet, recommends the National Health Service (NHS) in England. Triplets can be placed on their backs next to each other across the bassinet if there is enough room.

If you choose separate bassinets, put them next to each other so your babies are close and can comfort each other. If you choose bassinets with mesh siding, they will be able to see each other.

Remember that getting into a bedtime routine will help your multiples get the message it's time to go to sleep. Choose the best routine for you, but it usually includes a bath, a change into pajamas, a feeding, and soothing music or white noise. Be sure to dim the lights, keep the room cool, and speak softly. Swaddling (securely wrapping each baby in a blanket) also helps your babies feel like they're in the womb and helps them to go to sleep.

Our boys were in their own cribs from day one. With twins, night feedings were a production that was easier to do in their room. My boys now love their room and are extremely happy when it's time to go in their cribs.

—*Andrea Orr, MD, a mom of 10-month-old twin boys and a pediatrician with Northwest Pediatrics Washington University Clinical Associates, in St. Louis, MO*

When to Call Your Doctor: Nighttime Waking

Newborns get up every couple of hours to eat. In fact, during the first couple of weeks, you should wake up your babies every three to four hours to eat if they haven't woken up on their own.

By the time your babies have reached two to three months old, they should begin sleeping five to six hours at a time, although not every baby falls in step no matter how much you might plead.

Call your doctor if you're concerned about your babies waking at night, especially if they're also not gaining weight at the pace they should, refusing to feed, producing fewer than four wet diapers a day, or having fewer bowel movements.

Also be on the lookout and call your doctor if you notice signs of sleep apnea, which include snoring, trouble breathing during sleep, sleepiness during the day, and behavior changes.

At first, the twins slept side by side in the same crib. Later, as they got bigger, we used two separate ones. We also used the Baby Shusher, a device that mimics the sounds heard in the womb, which helped soothe them to sleep.

—*Saira Butt, MD, a mom of three-year-old twins and an infectious diseases physician, in Carmel, IN*

Sleep is huge for my husband and me, so we started a sleep routine as early as possible. When our boys first came home, we started bedtime at between 8 and 9 p.m., and we progressively moved it earlier as they began establishing better sleep habits.

—*Andrea Orr, MD*

DR. SONAL'S TIPS

For my twins' first few months, my mom was staying with us. At first, everyone was so eager to help that we all got up each time the babies woke. But in no time, we all were exhausted.

To get more sleep, my husband and my mother slept in shifts so they each got four to five hours of uninterrupted sleep a night. My mom stayed up for the first shift while my husband slept in the extra bed in the nursery, and then they swapped. Meanwhile I slept in between feedings.

People like to tell you to "nap when your baby naps." That sounds great, but this is hard with twins because they often nap at different times. When my girls napped at different times or when they napped for only 30 minutes, there was no time for me to nap as well.

Luckily for me, having gone through medical residency, I'm used to being sleep deprived. I can function well despite sleep deprivation.

In hindsight, I wish my husband and I had more help, especially at night. If we had gotten more sleep, we would have been less stressed.

When my boys were babies, I was a stickler with their schedule. If one woke up to eat, I woke the other up too and fed them both, changed them both, and put them both back to bed.

Sometimes I'd change the first baby, then wake the other, take him to my husband, and wake him up and say, "Your baby's ready to go." We'd take both babies to the living room and feed them together.

> —*Amy J. Lynch, DO, a mom of eight-year-old twin boys and a five-year-old son and a physical medicine and rehabilitation specialist at the Iowa Clinic, in Des Moines*

HEATHER'S TIPS

My wonderful family, friends, husband, and the Internet (LOL) really helped me through the first year of parenting twins. I always enjoyed searching for tips and suggestions online during my new schedule/free time (3 a.m., 5 a.m., etc.), and I wanted to share two of my favorite pieces of advice.

1. "Don't let other people's advice worry/bother you. Most people had only one baby at a time. It's much different with two! Never feel like a bad parent because you aren't doing what parents of singletons are (whatever it may be)."

I love that advice from Babble (Babble.com) because it came to me on a day I needed to hear it. So many people told

MommyTime

Take Advantage of an Early Bedtime

I would put my twins to sleep earlier so I would have a couple of hours before bedtime to relax. I'd spend the time with my spouse—or sleep myself.

—Saira Butt, MD

me how many places they visited or what they did the first year they were parents, but as a new mom to twins, doing those outings seemed impossible. Over time I learned that it is hard for parents of singletons to truly understand. Their advice is based on their experiences, and the intricacies of having two are not accounted for, but I learned over the next two years I would be able to do all those outings and more!

2. "There's no right way to do it. The best advice only works half the time. And Mom, it's not your fault."

I love this advice as well from Laura (SunnyDayFamily.com) because it is the truth! I always searched online hoping to find and solve all my struggles (getting both my boys to sleep through the night or getting them to eat vegetables). It became frustrating when the recommended solutions didn't work, and I always felt guilty. But over time I learned you can't rush things. It will happen eventually.

Before I had my twins, I was advised to wake up the other twin in the middle of the night as soon as one of them wakes to feed. While I think this is good advice for the first few months, be ready to reconsider if this means waking up your other twin unnecessarily.

When my twins were about four months old, I noticed that my son was always waking up first. I would feed him and then wake up his sister for her feeding. One day I realized that she might sleep through the night if she wasn't woken up, and sure enough she did, most nights. We still had to wake up with our son, but at least we had only one baby to take care of instead of two during the middle of the night.

—*Valerie Sheppard, MD, a mom of five-year-old boy/girl twins and a pediatrician with Newport Children's Medical Group, in Newport Beach, CA*

Because our twins were preemies, we had a night nanny until they were seven months old and could be sleep trained. The night nanny was at our home from 10 p.m. to 6 a.m. This saved our lives. Literally.

This isn't an option for everyone, but maybe a relative or friend could pitch in some nights.

—*Leah Cobb, MD, a mom of 20-month-old twins and a pediatric orthopedic surgeon at San Jorge Children's Hospital, in San Juan, PR*

My twins were adopted, so I didn't take maternity leave. We brought them home on the weekend, and I was back to work on Thursday.

Because I needed to be alert at work, not sleep deprived, we hired a night nurse. At $50 an hour, we quickly realized that was overkill for someone to feed healthy babies each night at 2 a.m.

Instead we hired a pre-nursing student. She stayed at our home each night from 10 p.m. to 6 a.m. She studied most of the night, and we gave her free use of the kitchen. She fed them each night for about six weeks until they began sleeping longer stretches at night. She was a lifesaver.

Later, we extended her hours to 8:30 a.m. so my husband and I had some time each morning to have a conversation.

—*Brooke A. Jackson, MD, a mom of 11-year-old twin girls and a 9-year-old son, a dermatologist, and the founder and medical director of the Skin Wellness Dermatology Associates, in Durham, NC*

Fast Facts

Mothers of multiples are more likely to be impacted by sleep deprivation. Only 14 percent of mothers of multiples get six or more hours of sleep per night in the first year.

For naps, I'd lie on my stomach under their Rock 'n Plays so they couldn't see me, one arm on each bar, and rock until they settled down. When they were small, my husband could carry one in each arm and sway back and forth until they fell asleep. All of this sounds like madness now. After some brief sleep training, they have slept through the night since they were about eight months old!

> —*Megan Lemay, MD, a mom of a three-year-old son and 22-month-old twin boys and an assistant professor of internal medicine at the Virginia Commonwealth University School of Medicine, in Richmond*

The books all tell you to "sleep when the baby sleeps." That sounds great, but for goodness' sakes, you have to do the laundry sometime!

> —*Brooke A. Jackson, MD*

DR. SONAL'S TIPS

Diaper changing at night is a challenge. If you're changing diapers, you're not sleeping! Generally, we changed our twins' diapers after they ate. A challenge was if they fell asleep feeding. Then I didn't want to wake them up. They were sensitive sleepers, and it could be hard to get them to go back to sleep. Yet I also didn't want to leave them in dirty diapers.

This caused me to change our routine. For a while, we changed their diapers before the nighttime feedings, instead of after. This had the added benefit of helping them wake up more to eat. The key is to be flexible with your routine as the babies' needs change.

❧

We established a very easy sleep routine. Every night we changed their diapers, put them into their sleep sacks, and then nursed them and put them directly into bed.

I don't feel that bathing them every night is beneficial, especially because my twins have a tendency to have dry skin. We don't add bath time to our bedtime routine. As they get older, we will add a book before bed and include their older sister in the process.

—*Meredith Brauer, MD, a mom of a three-year-old daughter and six-month-old boy-girl twins and an internal medicine hospitalist at Central DuPage Hospital, in Winfield, IL*

❧

We never rocked our twins to sleep. Some experts say that rocking babies to sleep regularly makes them dependent on the action because they learn to associate the rocking with sleep.

Experts often advise putting the baby in her crib "drowsy but awake." Personally, I think this is a pipe dream.

Our bedtime ritual was bath, bottle, story, bed. Usually, the twins fell asleep with the bottle.

—*Leah Cobb, MD*

By the time my twins were two months old, their bedtime routine was an essential part of our lives. Nightly baths started at 6:30 p.m., followed by a gentle lotion rub. Then we put them in their pajamas. We followed that with their nighttime bottle and then read them a book.

While we do our boys' bedtime routine, we use a white noise machine on low and dim the lights. Once feeding and reading time are over, we put each baby in his own crib in a sleep sack. We turn the white noise machine on high and turn out the lights.

—*Andrea Orr, MD*

DR. SONAL'S TIPS

To help the twins sleep, we used white noise in the nursery. Our house can be loud, and this way, we didn't have to be so quiet. Plus, the girls' movements and noises in their sleep would sometimes wake each other up. When the twins were younger, we used a Cloud B stuffed animal that played soothing sounds. As they got older, we used a HEPA air filter instead, which doubled as a white noise machine.

For the first four months, my girls slept in a co-sleeper in our room. Then they moved to cribs in the nursery. For a while they shared a crib because they were small enough and liked sleeping together. We separated them to their own cribs when they were around eight months old, when they started rolling around and bumping into each other.

As our twins got older, we did a little sleep training—letting them cry a bit before going to get them. As they started to indicate they could sleep longer, I tried to stretch out the times between feedings.

—*Amy J. Lynch, DO*

We sleep trained our twins when they were nine months old. Sleep training will be more difficult with twins because they will feed off of each other. Hang in there! It will eventually get better!

—*Valerie Sheppard, MD*

My husband and I focused as much as we could on putting our twins in their cribs to nap, rather than holding them or using baby swings. When our twins met the requirements— roughly weighing eight pounds each and consuming a minimum of 24 ounces of milk in a 24-hour period—we used the *Twelve Hours' Sleep by Twelve Weeks Old* book/method for sleep training, and it truly worked well for us. While I realize this isn't the case for everyone, we had great results.

—*Anne Rodrigue, DO, a mom of two-year-old twin girls and an ob-gyn at Thibodaux Women's Center, in Louisiana*

When our twins were seven months old, we sleep trained, letting them cry it out. They slept through the night from then on. We took away their pacifiers at seven months when we began training, and this seemed to be the key to success.

—*Leah Cobb, MD*

Dr. Sonal's Tips

When they were around 18 months old, we let our twins cry it out to learn to go to sleep. I wish we had done it sooner. My husband and I got our nanny on board for this. You need to have everyone on the same page. Because our nanny was so soft-hearted, I knew she would have a hard time listening to them cry. So I chose a time to do this when I'd be home for a few days straight.

When I sleep trained my girls, I put them in their cribs, gave them their blankets, said good night, and walked out of the room. Yes, they cried. A lot. My husband and I took turns wearing earplugs! We didn't both wear them in case of emergency. It took only a week or two before they would fall asleep peacefully on their own.

༺⚬ঌ

One thing that was critical when my twins were babies was sleep training. We used the Dr. Weissbluth method, which is explained in his book *Healthy Sleep Habits, Happy Child*. It's the "sleep bible" in my house.

My babies started teething right around three months, which was when we began sleep training. My husband did most of the sleep training because I couldn't stand the screaming. The first night, the twins screamed for an hour, but the next night it was 57 minutes, and it was less each night. They were sleep trained in about a week. Then we had our life back.

—*Brooke A. Jackson, MD*

Growing up, my twin and I had to share a room. We didn't like that.

When my twins were babies, they slept in separate cribs in the same room. They didn't seem to wake each other up. But they didn't offer any comfort to each other either!

My boys each have their own bedroom now. That's going well. Even though they have their own rooms, they often choose to sleep in the same room. That closeness is special.

—*Amy J. Lynch, DO*

Our twins have always shared a room. When we lived in our townhouse in Chicago, the master suite was on the first floor. We kept the baby monitor on until the girls were seven years old because they were so funny. My husband and I loved listening to their conversations. Plus, if they were crying, we knew right away and could go help.

Even now, my girls are still in the same room. When we moved to our current house in North Carolina, we tried to separate them, giving them each their own room. They originally said they wanted their own rooms. That lasted for two nights. Then they started sleeping in the same room again. Five years later, they're still sleeping there.

—*Brooke A. Jackson, MD*

Mommy MD Guides–Recommended Product
Fisher-Price Rock 'n Play Sleeper

Here's a product that helps your child fall asleep and allows you to get some sleep or free time for yourself as well. It has two settings of auto-rocking: one for naptime and one for nighttime. It also plays music and nature sounds so you can customize it to find just the right settings for your babies. Plus, it folds easily so you can store it or take it with you when you travel. The pad is removable and machine washable. What more could you ask for?

You can buy the Fisher-Price Rock 'n Play Sleeper at **FISHER-PRICE.MATTEL.COM** for $79.99.

MomMy TIME

Hire a Babysitter for *Your* Naps

It's not at all surprising to hear that mothers of multiples are significantly sleep deprived and experience symptoms of depression. In one study, mothers of eight-week-old twins were getting less than six hours of sleep a night.

Sleep deprivation isn't something to power through. Chronic sleepiness makes it hard to concentrate and make decisions, and it can lead to long-term health problems, such as high blood pressure, diabetes, and heart disease. Plus, drowsiness can result in a serious accident while you're driving or at home.

If friends and neighbors have offered to babysit, invite them to come over in the afternoon. Instead of heading out the door, sneak off to your bedroom for a nap (with earplugs if needed). Even better, make a daily appointment with your pillow. Hire a babysitter from a website such as **CARE.COM** or **SITTERCITY.COM**. You and your babies will be healthier when you practice self-care and you'll be setting a great example.

Chapter 5

Coping with Health Challenges

Multiples have shared everything since they were in the womb. Unfortunately, that also includes germs when they're sick. And they will get sick. Children under the age of two tend to get 8 to 10 colds a year, according to the American Academy of Pediatrics.

The first thing to do when one baby gets sick is to put the kibosh on sharing. Don't let your babies share pacifiers, toys, bottles, or sippy cups. You may want to separate them into different rooms at night. This is also the time to practice frequent hand washing for both you and your multiples and stay on top of sanitizing toys (throw them in the dishwasher if you can) and wash bedding in hot water.

It's okay to break from your usual routine and let your sick baby rest. Be sure your baby is drinking enough and continues to produce wet diapers. Be on the lookout for signs of a more serious illness. See the "When to Call Your Doctor" box on page 54 to know when your baby's symptoms call for a visit to the pediatrician or the hospital.

You can relieve a baby's stuffy nose by using a suction bulb and help your baby breathe by using a cool-mist humidifier. Acetaminophen and ibuprofen can help with a fever, but consult your doctor before giving it to a child younger than two, and call your doctor right away if your baby is younger than three months old and has a fever.

And as you're taking care of everyone else, remember to keep yourself healthy. Get enough sleep (if possible) and eat well.

The rest of the time, focus on prevention. Everyone in the family, including children six months and older, should get a flu vaccine every year. If your babies are less than three months old, ask friends and family members not to visit if they have a cold. Also teach older children to sneeze into their elbow or a tissue, which gets thrown away immediately.

Fast Facts

If one twin is hospitalized for RSV (respiratory syncytial virus), the other twin has a 34 percent chance of also being hospitalized with bronchiolitis, according to research published in the *Israel Medical Association Journal*.

Our twins had Twin to Twin Transfusion Syndrome (TTTS), which is a disease of the placenta that can affect identical twin pregnancies when twins share a common placenta. The twins were born at 34 weeks due to a heart problem in the bigger twin due to the TTTS.

I was on bed rest from 18 weeks on, and honestly, I did not cope well at all—lots of crying, worrying, and reading every bit of literature on TTTS I could find. Luckily, we all came out okay. Both twins survived and are healthy.

Being stuck on bed rest for months in a Puerto Rican hospital with no WiFi or TV was really hard. I really wanted a visit from my dog and my friends from back home in Alabama, but no one was able to make the trip. One of my friends sent a long text every few days, and this was an enormous help.

My husband was a total rock, but I could have used a lot more support than people were able to provide.

Our twins got early intervention physical therapy for about six months, but now, happily, all seems to be normal.

—*Leah Cobb, MD, a mom of 20-month-old twins and a pediatric orthopedic surgeon at San Jorge Children's Hospital, in San Juan, PR*

Fast Facts

Identical twins do not have the same dental records. Twins might start teething at the same time, but the shape of their teeth and how they are positioned will be different.

Our twins were born at 34 weeks, and both of them stayed in the NICU for 19 days. They needed to be fed through NG tubes (a feeding tube inserted through the nose) because they had immature feeding patterns. As they grew, they both learned to feed normally.

—*Andrea Orr, MD, a mom of 10-month-old twin boys and a pediatrician with Northwest Pediatrics Washington University Clinical Associates, in St. Louis, MO*

My twins were born at 36 weeks. They had some respiratory and feeding problems at first, but thankfully nothing life threatening. They were in the NICU for eight days, and I never imagined how hard this would be for me emotionally.

As a pediatrician who trained in the NICU, I assumed that if I knew their lives weren't in danger and they were getting stronger each day, I'd be okay with them needing and receiving NICU care. Instead, I was an emotional wreck! My maternal instincts took over the doctor side of my brain, and I wanted my babies home with me right away.

To other parents with twins in the NICU I'd like to say: Being a NICU parent probably will not be like anything you imagined. Allow yourself to feel whatever you feel and try to stay positive. It can seem like an eternity until your babies are home with you.

—*Valerie Sheppard, MD, a mom of five-year-old boy/girl twins and a pediatrician with Newport Children's Medical Group, in Newport Beach, CA*

My boy twin ended up in the NICU for a week and a half to learn how to eat efficiently, which is very common for preemie boys. It was difficult having to be in two places at once, and I felt guilty about spending so much time with one twin and not the other once we were home.

But it was much harder on my husband! He felt as though he couldn't do anything to help either child because I was nursing. We enlisted the help of my mother-in-law, who took over caring for our oldest while the two of us went back and forth between the hospital and home to spend time with each of the twins. One of us was there for every one of his feedings during the day. It helped to get to know the nurses taking care of him because when I couldn't be there, I knew he was in good hands.

Ultimately, I kept telling myself that this was just a very short blip of time in our experience together. Now, nearly seven months later, that first two weeks is all just a blur. We tried not to get our hopes up every day thinking he might come home. I knew that the best place for him was to be in the NICU, and until he was really ready to come home, we wanted him to be well taken care of.

—Meredith Brauer, MD, a mom of a three-year-old daughter and six-month-old boy-girl twins and an internal medicine hospitalist at Central DuPage Hospital, in Winfield, IL

Both of our boys needed supplemental oxygen. One twin continued to need oxygen for 10 days after we brought them home.

We came home with a compressor and several oxygen tanks, and we had cords everywhere. We also needed a pulse oximetry machine (to measure blood oxygen levels), and it went off constantly, mostly when he was kicking or crying. We couldn't get the beeping noise out of our heads. We were ecstatic when he no longer needed the oxygen and we could send all the equipment back!

—*Andrea Orr, MD*

It's been very hard not to try to doctor my own kids, and I'm not even a pediatrician. One of my twins has a small head circumference (not discovered until after birth), and I have worried about him a lot. I can't stop myself from watching his milestones like a hawk. Luckily, he often hits them before his identical twin does!

I had to learn to trust their pediatrician and stop myself from reading research papers. You just cannot put them into context when it's your own kids.

—*Megan Lemay, MD, a mom of a three-year-old son and 22-month-old twin boys and an assistant professor of internal medicine at the Virginia Commonwealth University School of Medicine, in Richmond*

DR. SONAL'S TIPS

One of my girls had colic. Sometimes my husband and I were at our wit's end with the crying.

We tried everything we could think of to soothe her—the "5 Ss" (swaddle, hold her on her side, shush, swing, and suck), holding her in a quiet room, playing soothing music, and holding her and swaying. Sometimes we took her for a drive. Nothing seemed to help consistently.

Sometimes it helped to bundle her up and take her outside. I think the change of scenery and distraction helped sometimes, but not always. We would have tried anything.

The only thing that really helped was time. Our daughter finally stopping crying when she was around six months old.

୧∕୦

My youngest twin had some reflux. He would wake from a dead sleep with a horrible cry. His doctor prescribed Prilosec, which did the trick for a couple of months until my son grew out of the reflux.

—*Amy J. Lynch, DO, a mom of eight-year-old twin boys and a five-year-old son and a physical medicine and rehabilitation specialist at the Iowa Clinic, in Des Moines*

My girls had terrible allergies and snoring. They both needed to have their tonsils removed when they were four years old.

We scheduled them for back-to-back surgeries. The doctor said, "If you bring one home and the other sees her, you'll never get the other one to surgery."

—*Brooke A. Jackson, MD, a mom of 11-year-old twin girls and a 9-year-old son, a dermatologist, and the founder and medical director of the Skin Wellness Dermatology Associates, in Durham, NC*

One of my worst parenting nights ever happened when my twins were around five months old. Of course, it always happens when your spouse is out of town, and mine was.

One of my girls got sick, and then the other one did. As soon as one stopped throwing up, the other started. They vomited so many times that I changed their clothes and sheets multiple times. By morning, I had done six loads of laundry. By that point, I was on the floor laughing.

When you have children in general—and twins in particular—you have to have a sense of humor. There's a direct correlation between the number of children you have and the greater the sense of humor you need to have. You just have to let it go.

—*Brooke A. Jackson, MD*

DR. SONAL'S TIPS

My girls both used pacifiers. They started in the hospital. I think pacifiers are helpful for twins because it's challenging to soothe two babies at once if you're by yourself.

I decided to take the girls' pacifiers away at age one, which is the time when they start impacting dental health. I hid them in a bag in my closet away from the girls, the nanny, and my husband. I knew one of them would break down and give in to the girls. Our nanny was a sweet grandma-like person who didn't like to see the kids cry. The girls adjusted to paci-free life in a week or two. I was proud of them.

We were very fortunate and didn't have to deal with major health issues with our twins. The biggest issues we faced were minor gastrointestinal upset and eczema.

Because of the eczema, we switched them both to completely unscented lotions, detergents, and other products. This was in keeping with our policy of "when one needs something, the other gets it too."

—*Anne Rodrigue, DO, a mom of two-year-old twin girls and an ob-gyn at Thibodaux Women's Center, in Louisiana*

Sicknesses that would last a week in single babies last for a month with twins. Viruses bounce back and forth between them. Then a parent gets sick. Then it cycles back to the kids.

The best thing you can do when your twins are sick is give yourself extra TLC.

—*Brooke A. Jackson, MD*

Fast Facts

Do identical twins have identical voices? Some do and some do not, but they have similar voices. Vocal characteristics are related to the vocal folds (more commonly known as vocal cords) as well as the surrounding muscles and structures (such as the size of the larynx).

Genetics plays a part in determining the shape and size of these structures, but many other factors can affect them. Hormones (especially during puberty), environmental factors such as pollutants in the air, certain medications, and how much one uses one's voice (for example, a lot of singing, talking, and yelling) are all factors that can alter the shape and size of the vocal folds and surrounding structures, which in turn alter the characteristics of one's voice.

DR. SONAL'S TIPS

It's helpful to remember that it's your choice when and if you have visitors over. If your babies are premature, you may have to be careful about getting them sick. Even if your friends and family members are excited to come and visit, do it on your own schedule. You're not being rude; you're just making your children and yourself a priority.

After my girls were born, we knew that my mother would be staying with us to help out. My in-laws of course were very excited for their first granddaughters and wanted to visit right away. They live six hours away, so they stayed with us for a week. They arrived the same day that we came home from the hospital. It was a little stressful having both my mom and my husband's parents stay with us. Everybody wanted to be super helpful. They wanted to be polite and do things in the "right" way and kept asking me lots of questions, but that wasn't helpful to me.

Looking back, I wish I had staggered my family's visits and waited to have so many visitors until after my girls had better established their schedule.

When to Call Your Doctor: Missed Milestones

Keeping in mind your twins' adjusted birthdate, watch for meeting milestones. If you are concerned that your twins have missed a milestone, talk with your babies' pediatrician.

Chapter 6

Staying Safe

Parents with one baby have their hands full. You have two or more who can take off in every direction once they're mobile. Wandering kids can get into everything from cleaning supplies to electrical outlets, so babyproofing is a must.

Get a head start on making your home safe by babyproofing before your babies come home from the hospital because life may become too hectic as you care for your growing babies. Use safety straps to anchor dressers, bookcases, TVs, and any tall piece of furniture to the wall to prevent them from tipping; place covers on the electrical outlets; install window guards; choose cordless shades or tie the cords up high where kids can't reach them; place bumpers on the sharp edges of tables; secure cabinets with babyproof locks; get a childproof lock for the oven door; place covers on door knobs; and keep medications in a lockbox.

Another good idea is to keep a list of emergency numbers by the phone, including numbers for poison control (1-800-222-1222), your pediatrician, the fire department, the police department, your pharmacy, you and your spouse's cell phones and work phones, and relatives and neighbors. When your children are old enough, it's helpful to teach them your cell phone number, address, full name, and when and how to call 911.

Don't forget about the car seats. Because multiples have a tendency to come early, you should have them installed and ready to go long before your due date. Hospitals, fire departments, and police stations often have programs to check that they're installed properly.

When to Call Your Doctor: Falls

It doesn't take much for children learning to walk or exploring a playground to take a tumble. Most of the time the cure is a little TLC.

But falls can be serious if your child suffers a head injury. Call your doctor if your child has a headache for more than 24 hours after falling. Go to the emergency room if your child was knocked out for less than a minute or fell from a dangerous height.

Call 911 if your child becomes unconscious for longer than a minute, has a seizure, slurs her speech, has trouble walking, has trouble moving her neck, or is confused.

Dr. Sonal's Tips

With twins, you need to be extra vigilant because they have you outnumbered. You can't confine them to one area because one runs off and then the other goes in the opposite direction.

We did the standard babyproofing; my husband was in charge of this. We put plugs in the outlets and knob covers on the doors so they wouldn't get out.

One thing that happened a lot was when one fell and got hurt, I'd try to console her, but then the other one would start crying. Logic doesn't work here, even when I'd explain: "Do you see your sister is hurt, so I'm helping her?" All they see is, "You picked up my sister, so why aren't you doing that to me?" I would pick them both up or hug both. Even to this day, when one gets a cold pack, the other one goes and gets a sympathy boo-boo pack too. Consequently, we always keep multiple boo-boo packs in the freezer at all times. We usually have four in case two are thawed out!

∽

My husband and I didn't get much time to ourselves when our twins were babies! My husband's a fireman, and I'm an ER doctor, so we tried to make time. The most important thing we did was to get a nanny. That helped give us both some freedom, and we could relax knowing that our children were safe and well cared for.

—*Cassie Cole, MD, a mom of five-year-old twin girls and an emergency physician, in Hot Springs, AR*

Mommy MD Guides-Recommended Product
Nokire TV Strap Anti-Tip Child Safety Furniture Straps

For parental peace of mind, these mounting straps are essential for any household. These heavy-duty security straps come with mounting screws to attach the strap to the VESA holes on the back of your TV. The other end attaches to your TV stand or a wall, and the metal buckle is tightened to ensure a strong hold. You can buy them for $27.99 at **AMAZON.COM**.

HEATHER'S TIPS

Part of keeping the house safe for twins is keeping it as neat and tidy as possible. I always leave out my twins' favorite toys and keep them easily accessible. Other toys that are less played with are gathered and put into six different Tupperware containers. We call them surprise boxes. I keep them in a closet, and each day I bring out a new surprise box. It will contain toys, puzzles, and activities.

My boys find the items in the surprise box so much fun— even though they are filled with toys they barely played with when they were easily accessible. Putting the toys away makes them new again when they are brought out. It is a very fun tradition for us, and my boys love getting a surprise box. It also gives me a little free time every day, which is a wonderful thing.

Room-by-Room Baby Proofing
NURSERY SAFETY CHECKLIST

- Choose safe cribs—be wary of used cribs, especially ones with drop-down sides.
- Look for a label saying the crib meets the U.S. Consumer Product Safety Commission standards.
- Look for a Juvenile Products Manufacturers Association (JPMA) seal.
- Avoid cribs with attached dressers that your babies could later use to climb out.
- Look for slats that are close together; you shouldn't be able to slide a soda can between them.
- Avoid corner posts that your babies' clothes could get stuck on.
- Assemble the cribs carefully.
- Make sure all hardware is tightened securely.
- Keep the cribs away from windows and out of reach of window treatments.
- Buy firm mattresses.
- Don't use bumper pads, and keep blankets, pillows, and toys out of the babies' cribs.
- Don't use sleep positioners.
- Make sure the sheets fit snugly; never use an adult sheet.
- Choose pj's with no ties, buttons, or snaps that could come off or get entangled.

- Clear a path that allows you to get to the cribs and from the cribs to the changing table.
- Secure bookcases and dressers to the floor or wall.
- Inspect toys with care; make sure they don't have small parts.
- Buy a changing table with four side rails and a safety strap.
- Always use the safety strap when changing your babies, or change your babies on the floor.
- Wash your hands after changing your babies.
- Cover electrical outlets.
- Install a night-light so you can get to your babies in the dark.
- Wash new clothes before your babies wear them.
- Wash toys before use.

BATHROOM SAFETY CHECKLIST

- Turn down your home's water temperature to 120°F.
- Check the water temperature in your home by running the hot water, filling a mug, and checking it with a food thermometer.
- Consider installing an anti-scald device.
- Have a safe place to put one baby, such as a bouncer seat with a strap, while you bathe the other.
- Choose a baby bathtub with a high back or support to keep your baby's head up and with a slip-resistant cushion to keep your baby warm and secure.

- Put only enough water in the tub to cover your baby's legs.
- Make the tub less slippery with a mat or stickers.
- Put an absorbent mat next to the tub to cushion your knees and to soak up water.
- Don't use a bath seat.
- Use a water temperature gauge to check your baby's bathwater.
- Lock cabinets.
- Keep the toilet lid down and consider buying a toilet lock.
- Keep things in their original containers.
- Store medication safely out of reach.
- Consider buying a locking medication safe.
- Have an idea of your babies' weights in case you have to give medication.
- Read the dosage instructions for medication each and every time you give it to your babies.
- Use the dropper, cup, or spoon that came with the medication—not a teaspoon.
- Turn on a light before giving your babies medication.
- Never treat vitamins and medicine like candy.
- Check expiration dates on all medications you give.
- Put a whiteboard on your fridge or in your bathroom and record medications given.
- Dispose of medications correctly; check with your pharmacy or police department for information on proper disposal.

- Keep bath oils out of reach; they can damage your baby's lungs if inhaled.
- Move appliances back toward the wall and secure cords.
- Unplug appliances, such as hair dryers and curling irons.
- Cover water spigots.
- Consider a drain valve cover.
- Keep babies away from water knobs.
- Install ground fault circuit interrupters.
- Never ever leave your babies unattended!

KITCHEN SAFETY CHECKLIST
- Switch to less toxic cleaning products.
- Move dangerous cleaning products to higher, locked locations.
- Store products and foods in their original containers.
- Lock your cabinets, trash cans, oven, stove, fridge, and dishwasher.
- Load sharp items into the dishwasher points down.
- Keep the oven and dishwasher doors closed.
- Consider investing in a splatter guard for the stove.
- Move appliances to the back of counters and keep cords from dangling.
- Unplug appliances when they are not in use.
- Get in the habit of using the back burners on your stove and turn pot handles to the back.

- Identify where your babies are before carrying hot pots and beverages.
- Never carry your babies and hot foods or drinks.
- Use place mats instead of tablecloths.
- Don't allow your babies to chew on keys or remotes.
- Quickly pick small items up off of the floor.
- Keep salt away from your babies; just 1½ tablespoons can be toxic.
- Keep purses and bags out of reach.
- Install ground fault circuit interrupters.
- Make sure window treatments, such as mini-blind strings, aren't accessible.

DINING ROOM SAFETY CHECKLIST

- Before feeding your babies, wash your hands.
- Measure baby formula carefully.
- If there's a chance your home has lead pipes, always use cold water and run it for one minute.
- Never warm baby bottles in the microwave.
- Check formula expiration dates, and never use dented containers.
- Discard uneaten formula.
- Never borrow or buy a used breast pump.
- Bolt heavy furniture to the wall or floor.
- Replace the tablecloth with place mats.
- Never put a bouncer seat or Bumbo chair on top of a table.

- Look for a high chair with a wide, stable base.
- Choose a high chair with a removable tray that you can wash well and even place in the dishwasher.
- Ensure the high chair has a safety strap, ideally with a post that goes between the baby's legs.
- Put your babies' high chairs in a safe location away from window blinds.
- Store your babies' bibs, spoons, and bowls in a handy location.
- Teach your babies to wash hands often and well.
- Feed your babies slowly to avoid choking.
- Avoid giving your babies foods that could lodge in their throats: cheese cubes, candy, hot dogs, marshmallows, jelly beans, peanuts, popcorn, raisins, grapes, seeds, and raw veggies.
- Make sure window treatments, such as mini-blind strings, aren't accessible.

LIVING ROOM SAFETY CHECKLIST

- Create a safe space for your babies here, such as in a Pack 'n Play.
- Choose a swing with a wide base and safety straps.
- Always place baby seats and bouncers on the floor—never on a table.
- Don't let your babies sleep on your chest or on the sofa.

Schedule a Date Night

If you can get out for a date night with your hubby, you certainly should. Both parents of multiples suffer from more depression, anxiety, and stress compared to other parents, according to studies.

Take advantage of family members and friends who offer to babysit and head out for a night on the town, just the two of you. Dress up and go to a nice restaurant, or throw on jeans and head to a low-key local joint. Go bowling, play mini-golf, see a movie, or go for a walk in the park. Whatever you decide, take a few hours to decompress and enjoy one-on-one time.

- If your babies are having tummy time, always watch them carefully.
- Bolt heavy furniture to the wall or floor.
- Make sure your babies can't grab the TV; push it back or strap it down.
- Rather than having another changing table here, change your babies on the floor.
- Create another diaper-changing station here, with the products kept out of the reach of your babies.
- Fasten down throw rugs.
- Never run extension cords under rugs.
- Never strike a match while holding a baby or have candles burning nearby.

- Watch for plant leaves that have dropped and pick them up.
- Remove glass-topped tables.
- Soften hard edges and corners of furniture with padding.
- Remove any tables that could tip over.
- Move breakables to higher ground.
- Cover your fireplace with a door guard, and secure it with a heat-resistant gate.

BEDROOM/OFFICE SAFETY CHECKLIST

- Have a safe "landing place" for your babies, such as a bassinet.
- Install outlet covers.
- Place a night-light if you need it to get out of your room to your babies' rooms quickly.
- Keep your room clutter-free.
- Remove glass-topped tables.
- Soften hard edges and corners of furniture with padding.
- Remove any tables that could tip over.
- Move breakables to higher ground.
- Keep all alcohol locked up.
- Unplug the shredder.
- Make sure window treatments, such as mini-blind strings, aren't accessible.

GARAGE/WORKSHOP/GYM SAFETY CHECKLIST

- Have a safe "landing place" for your babies, especially if you ever have to work while your baby's here.
- Lock up any toxic chemicals.
- Consider power strip covers or place strips high.
- Keep lids securely on trash cans and recyclables cans.
- Test your garage door's two-second reverse mechanism.
- Store all tools out of reach in a locked closet or shed.
- Buy antifreeze that contains denatonium benzoate, which makes the sweet liquid taste bad.
- Put a door knob cover on the door to the workshop, garage, or workout room to keep babies out!

YARD SAFETY CHECKLIST

- Apply sunscreen 20 to 30 minutes before going outside.
- Reapply sunscreen every two to three hours.
- Protect your babies' eyes with sunglasses.
- Dress your babies in neutral colors, such as white and khaki, to keep insects away.
- Keep your babies' fingers and toes free and clear when opening and closing the stroller.
- Buckle your babies each and every time into the stroller, swing, etc.
- Keep the trash and recyclables cans covered.
- Store tools in a locked cabinet or shed.
- Add railing guards to balconies and decks.

- Keep furniture away from deck rails.
- Teach your babies to stay far away from grills.
- Install baby gates at the top of all deck stairs.
- Learn about the plants in your yard, and keep your babies away from sharp and/or poisonous ones.
- Pull out any fungi in your yard.
- Buy and plant only nontoxic plants and shrubbery.
- Don't use lawn chemicals.

Pilates

My time for myself was Pilates. I did it before pregnancy and beyond. I made time for it even when I did not have extra money; that is how important it was. I do not do massage, polish my nails, wear makeup, buy myself clothes, or travel. I thought caring for my body and mind will pay for itself rather than spending money on other goods or services.

Also, I cannot overstate enough the importance of time to sleep, especially the first year and beyond. Try to get enough sleep.

If you are like me, an introvert, then you might have to get used to noise and someone somewhere crying all the time, and learn for ways to cope. I like spending time in nature too and taking the kids with me. Nature and classical music also help in my case to calm both me and the kids.

—Maria Peters, MD, a mom of five-year-old
boy/girl twins and an ophthalmologist
in private practice in Los Angeles, CA

Chapter 7

Fostering Personality

People are fascinated by twins and multiples, especially if they're identical. Often people focus on the similarities, from hair and eye color to mannerisms and speaking in sync. But the truth is that your children are individuals with distinctive personalities. Establishing their own identity will allow them to build their sense of self, which helps with their development and makes them more confident and better able to deal with challenges. And as they get older, they'll be more open to change if you don't dress and treat them the same when they're young.

Experts also say that when multiples develop their own identity, it helps with their social and language skills and lessens competition and fighting. Plus, it decreases separation anxiety and encourages healthier relationships with others.

You can foster their unique identities by letting them be individuals. Start by calling them by their names rather than referring to them as "the twins." Also help others recognize them as individuals. Dress them for playdates in different clothes. Send them to day care or preschool with different haircuts or wearing their favorite (different) colors.

At home, let them choose their own snacks, read them their bedtime stories separately, give them different gifts for their birthdays (and even separate cakes or birthday parties), sing happy birthday to each child separately, allow them to each choose what to wear, take pictures of each alone instead of always together, give them their own space, and encourage them to make their own friends. You can encourage family members to do the same.

It's also a great idea for you and your spouse to spend time with each child one-on-one. Set a timer and focus on playing with or reading to one child. Then set the timer for another child so each knows they will get their own special time with you. At dinner, ask each child individually to tell you about their day. Also take time for a special lunch date with one of your kids one week, then do the same with the other child the next week.

And as your twins get older, their individual interests will become more obvious. One twin boy may like music, while the other likes building Legos. Pay attention to these differences and encourage them to follow their own interests.

Sometimes multiples struggle to express their own feelings when they are different from those of other siblings. You could show them pictures of children and explain that one child likes art while another likes sports, and that's perfectly fine.

It's also okay for them to want to do activities together or dress similarly, but let them know they have a choice. Most importantly, let each child know you love and respect him or her.

DR. SONAL'S TIPS

Once my husband and I learned we were having girls, we chose their names. We didn't want the twins' names to match. We felt it was important for each girl to have her own unique sense of identity. We wanted them to feel different from each other—not to be always lumped together in a set.

My husband and I each came up with a list of names independently. Then we exchanged lists and ranked each other's lists: first favorite, second favorite, etc. We asked our family and friends for some input, and then we picked the top names from each list.

Our families are from India. Some Indian names are difficult for Americans to pronounce, so we were careful to avoid those names. We didn't want the girls' names to be butchered in school. I knew some of my family was disappointed that we didn't pick more traditional names.

In our culture, it's traditional for a baby's middle name to be the father's first name. So our girls share the same middle name.

We chose our daughters' names before they were born, but we didn't tell anyone else until they were born. We wanted their names to be a surprise.

My husband made T-shirts for the grandparents and our siblings. He gave them when they visited, and we wore them for a photo. It was our first "welcome home" family photo. The T-shirts said, "Welcome, Maya and Sophia!"

As my girls were growing, I kept a journal on the desktop of my computer. My office is next to their bedroom, so it was easy for me to go in and work on it when they were sleeping.

In the journal I kept track of "firsts" and milestones and funny things my girls did and said. If you don't write the details down, you forget them. It's especially difficult keeping these details straight with twins.

—*Brooke A. Jackson, MD, a mom of 11-year-old twin girls and a 9-year-old son, a dermatologist, and the founder and medical director of the Skin Wellness Dermatology Associates, in Durham, NC*

My twins are nine years old. This is the first year they wanted to have separate birthday parties. Truth be told, we haven't had many birthday parties. We did a combined party for both twins when they were in first grade.

This year, they wanted separate parties so they could each invite their own friends. My daughter had hers at Sky Zone, and my son had his at a rock climbing gym.

—*Jennifer Gilbert, DO, a mom of nine-year-old boy-girl twins and an ob-gyn at Paoli Hospital, in Pennsylvania*

Fast Facts
Dogs are able to tell identical twins apart, partly due to individual odors that each twin has.

DR. SONAL'S TIPS

Now that our girls are older, to foster each twin's unique personality, we do a variety of things. We sing "Happy Birthday" twice so they each get their moment of individual attention.

My sister likes to bake, so she bakes each girl her own birthday cake. This way they don't have to share. She lets them choose what flavor of cake they want and how they want it to be decorated.

When the opportunity allows, especially now that they are older, I let the girls choose their own style and color of shoes, lunchbox, backpack, etc.

One of our girls is left-handed—in our otherwise right-handed family. This makes her unique and special, but we are all adjusting trying to teach her how to write and do things left-handed. We try to celebrate this uniqueness about her.

As my girls have grown, I saved some of their onesies and other special clothes and bibs. I had a quilt made for each of them. I'm going to give the quilts to them when they're old enough to keep them safe.

༄

As twins grow, it's fascinating to learn their unique characteristics. One of my girls is the "rule follower"; the other is more "go with the flow."

With discipline, I learned the best approach is to determine what it is they really enjoy and withdraw that. For instance, we will take away screen time.

—*Brooke A. Jackson, MD*

A challenge I sometimes have with my twins is when one needs help with something but the other doesn't. Sometimes they lapse into taunting each other: "You don't know how to do that? It's sooo easy."

I try to help them rise above that. Instead I focus on positive reinforcement, saying things like, "You're doing a good job. Let's practice. Stay positive."

—*Jennifer Gilbert, DO*

My girls argue all of the time. Some of it is age appropriate, such as when they were little, they argued over toy snatching.

One of the things twins have way too much of is sharing. They know how to share, but it can be difficult for them to have to share everything all of the time, especially when there's another sibling who doesn't have to share as much.

—*Brooke A. Jackson, MD*

Fast Facts

Twins live longer than singletons, and their close social connection may be a major reason why. Researchers studied more than 2,900 same-sex twins who were born in Denmark between 1870 and 1900. The researchers compared the twins to the general Danish population. At every age, identical twins had higher survival rates than fraternal twins. And fraternal twins had higher survival rates than people in the general population.

I think it would be easy for twins to compete with each other all of the time. Fortunately, it's not my twins' nature to be competitive. My husband and I have always stopped competition right away and redirected them. We'll say things like, "You are really good at this. Sometimes it takes a little longer to do that. It took me longer too. You're like Mommy."

They do compare each other, though. I try to find things that they each excel at, to remind them of their strengths. It's key at this age for their confidence that they have a skill set they know, that they can rely on. So they can think, *I'm good at this.*

—*Jennifer Gilbert, DO*

DR. SONAL'S TIPS

I think it's important to have one-on-one time with each of my girls. My husband and I used to be better about it. We tried every few weeks to spend time with the children individually. For example, my husband would take one to the park while I stayed home and played with the other child. The next weekend we switched off. This way, each child got to spend some alone time with each parent.

My husband and I work hard to foster a sense of collaboration, of peace, between our twins. When they do something unkind to each other, we call them out right away by saying, "That's not nice. That might have hurt your twin's feelings. How would you feel if someone did that to you?"

Also, my husband and I model kindness toward each other. It matters how you interact with your partner. Watch your words; use kind words. Kids really see that.

—*Jennifer Gilbert, DO*

One thing parents of multiples find hard is that you spread yourself really thin. Before our third child was born, my husband and I took turns having "princess dates" where he took one twin out and I took the other. Our twins really valued that alone time with us.

—*Brooke A. Jackson, MD*

Fast Facts

By studying twins, scientists were able to determine that most personality traits are inherited. When scientists compared the personality traits of twins who were raised together against those who were raised apart, they found that the personalities of twins who were raised apart were more similar than they expected. The researchers concluded that personality traits are mostly determined by genetics. Interestingly, the traits most strongly determined by heredity are leadership and obedience to authority.

I try to do one-on-one time with each of my boys. They have a little brother now, and I'm often with him while my husband is with the twins. He coaches their sports. If he's taking one twin to an activity, then I'm with the other one.

I take advantage of this time to focus on him alone. That's really important.

Now that my twins are older, they're better at asking for and getting what they need. If I'm alone reading a book, one of them will usually come to me and hang out with me.

—Amy J. Lynch, DO, a mom of eight-year-old twin boys and a five-year-old son and a physical medicine and rehabilitation specialist at the Iowa Clinic, in Des Moines

When to Call Your Doctor: Twin Separation Anxiety

Experts say it's important as a parent to encourage your multiples to be individuals, with their own friends and experiences. However, it's completely normal for multiples to have some anxiety about being separated from their siblings. Be understanding about their separation anxiety as you gently encourage them to spend some time apart, whether on a special outing with a parent or in separate classrooms if you think that's right for them.

If your children are having a lot of difficulty being separated, consider talking to a psychologist who has experience with multiples. A psychologist can help you understand your children's relationship and guide your multiples on how to feel less anxious when they're not together.

DR. SONAL'S TIPS

I think a lot about the importance of treating twins equally. Everyone tries to do their best, but this won't always work out. And it doesn't have to. You have to look at each child's individual needs. Treating each one the same is not always a benefit. There will be fights about this, and there will be sibling rivalry. But I emphasize to my girls that they are their own person.

For example, when they were younger, one daughter fell and was crying, so I was holding her and helping her. Then the other one started bawling, asking, "Why are you hugging her and not me?"

I told them it's like medicine. If one is sick and has to take medicine, but the other is not sick, that doesn't mean I should give the not-sick one medicine. When they were babies, one twin had eczema, so we had to put oatmeal in her bath. I remember my father-in-law asking me why I didn't put oatmeal in her sister's bath too. First, she didn't need it for her skin. Second, it causes a sticky, gooey mess that I'd have to clean up after each bath, which would have created more work for me. Plus, I'd have to keep running to the store to get more bath oats. Not doing everything exactly the same for each child doesn't make you a bad mother.

MomMy TIME

Take a Coffee Break and Read a Magazine

Sometimes it's the little things that help you through the day, such as taking 15 minutes to sip a cup of coffee and page through a magazine (or read celebrity gossip online if that's more your thing). Try to take these precious minutes every day during naptime or when your babies are happy and safe in their cribs or Pack 'n Plays. Taking time for you is an essential part of self-care.

In the past, people tended to buy the same gifts, clothes, and toys for twins, thinking they would not want to share but would want the same things. Today, parents are encouraged to highlight the differences between siblings. The feeling is to not have them share everything, because they always share the most important thing—their parents.

A great step toward this is to label each child's items so that both you and the child come to know what belongs to each one. NameBubbles specializes in waterproof labels that stand up to laundry and dishwashing. They offer tons of personalizations, from colors to logos to name fonts, to suit each child's personality. The number of products they offer is incredible—labels for clothes, bottles, day care essentials, and anything else you can think of. Go to **NAMEBUBBLES.COM** for a list of products and prices as well as a video that shows just how well their labels stand up to daily use.

HEATHER'S TIPS

It can be hard for friends and even family members to tell your twins apart. Sharing ways to identify your twins can help people get to know each of them, and it encourages individuality for your twins. Some ideas are:

- *Buy your twins different shoes and socks.*
- *Write their names on the sole of their shoes where others can see it.*
- *Have them pick different hairstyles or haircuts.*
- *Or the classic: Have them wear different colors.*

It is important for twins to see themselves as two unique individuals rather than a unit or as "the twins." It can also be a safety measure too. Imagine you are at a family party and one of your twins reaches up for the hot stove. If your family member or other surrounding adults cannot yell their name to get their attention, an accident could happen. Not providing tips to help identify your twins can also lead people to come up with identifiers of their own. Several twin parents and even I have had people say things like: he/she is the bigger one, the happier one, the more athletic one . . . and those identification practices can be hurtful to twins as they get older.

Chapter 8:

Going to School and Work

Life has been hectic since you brought your multiples home from the hospital. Now there will be new challenges to adjust to. If you're going back to work, your mornings are getting busier as you get yourself ready for work and your babies ready for day care or even a nanny coming to your house. It's probably easiest if you set your alarm to get up, take a shower, do your hair and makeup, and eat breakfast before getting your babies up to change and feed them. Some moms wait until they're about to walk out the door to put on their work clothes to avoid spit-up stains.

Many moms of twins make things a little easier on themselves by bringing at least a week of supplies to day care to avoid having to worry about it every morning. You can ask your center if you can drop off a box of formula and a case of diapers and wipes for them to use until they run out. You can also keep several extra outfits at day care so they're there if needed. It also helps to have your bag packed for day care the night before so you can grab it and go in the morning.

It's always hard to leave your little ones when it's time to head back to work, but there are some pluses to this change. For one, you'll have adult interaction and conversation again, which is a biggie if you have felt isolated since having your multiples. Some moms also say day care helped their babies get into a daily routine of sleeping, eating, and playing.

Or maybe your new challenge is sending your little ones to school. If that's the case, the biggest question you may have is whether or not to put them in the same classroom. There is no one-size-fits-all answer to this question, but researchers who have looked into it agree on one thing: It's a decision that should be made based on the wishes of the parents, teachers—and the kids. Unfortunately, one study by a California researcher found that too often schools set a policy of separating twins and that some principals believe the twins will perform better academically, but that hasn't been found to be true. In a study that looked at twins in Canada and the United Kingdom, the researchers found that separating them had neither a positive or negative effect on their academic achievement.

Fast Facts

Twenty-two percent of twins are left-handed. The number is just under 10 percent for singletons.

DR. SONAL'S TIPS

I took six months off after my twins were born. I am so grateful that my employer let me do that. I told myself I should because most people take two to three months with just one baby. I thought, Why shouldn't I take off six months with two babies?

Before my twins were born, I brought home a bag full of work. I didn't look at that bag once. I have no regrets. I didn't have time, and even if I did have time, I still wouldn't have worked.

When it was time for me to go back to work, I went back full-time. Not everyone has this luxury, I know. I was fortunate, and that really helped my sanity. I switched to part-time when the girls were three years old.

One thing that I didn't do, that I wish I had done, was to have the nanny speak Spanish to the children. One of my friends had her nanny speak in Spanish, and her kids learned how to speak Spanish before entering school. Bilingual language development is great for early brain development. Today my girls are in a dual-language immersion program learning Spanish.

My twins were in the same kindergarten class. It was full-day kindergarten. I noticed my daughter was hovering over my son. She kept telling him what to do!

Before first grade, I talked with the principal. She agreed it would be best to split them up. That turned out to be the best decision. They could develop their own friendships and grow as individuals.

—*Jennifer Gilbert, DO, a mom of nine-year-old boy-girl twins and an ob-gyn at Paoli Hospital, in Pennsylvania*

Dr. Sonal's Tips

When my girls went to preschool and transitional kindergarten, they were in the same classroom. We didn't choose that; the schools had only one class in those grade levels. Having their sister in class with them helped them adjust to school and eased their separation anxiety.

Now that my girls are in kindergarten, I chose to have them in separate classes. My girls have very different personalities and learning styles, and I felt it was important for them to develop their individuality.

In the coming years, we'll see how this plays out. My cousin, who has older twins, said she had her twins initially together, then separate, then back together. I can imagine that having two separate sets of homework, two open houses to go to, two Christmas parties, multiple Christmas presents for teachers, and inviting 50 classmates over to a birthday party all become a little bit too much.

HEATHER'S TIPS

The days are long, but the years are very short. Enjoy and celebrate each milestone. I cherish every memory with my twins, and each moment is forever saved in my heart.

Watching twins grow and seeing their close bond is incredible. I asked my twins, "What do you like about being a twin?" and I wanted to share their answers: Gavin said, "The best thing is always having someone who has your back and sticks up for you." Grant said, "The best thing about being a twin is that I always have someone to help me and be my best friend." Being a parent of twins has beautiful days and hard days. Just remember you can do it.

Consider Hiring a Part-Time Nanny

Recently, we hired a nanny from 4 p.m. to 8 p.m. She takes care of our twins after school for a little bit, and I can go to the gym. She cooks and cleans and helps put them to bed with us so my husband and I don't have to do anything except spend time with each other after they go to sleep. Godsend. Before we had the nanny, I had no time to myself.

—Leah Cobb, MD, a mom of 20-month-old twins
and a pediatric orthopedic surgeon
at San Jorge Children's Hospital, in San Juan, PR

Early on, when my twins were in day care, they mainly played with each other. However, they tended to get in trouble more often when they played together.

So when we were getting ready to send them to kindergarten, my husband and I requested they be in separate classrooms. Their behavior is better when they're not together.

Now they each have their own friends. They have some shared friends, but mainly they each have separate friends.

—*Amy J. Lynch, DO, a mom of eight-year-old twin boys and a five-year-old son and a physical medicine and rehabilitation specialist at the Iowa Clinic, in Des Moines*

When to Call Your Doctor: Learning Disability

If your child is struggling with reading or writing, it doesn't mean she isn't as smart as other children who pick it up quickly. It only means your child learns differently. This may be more common in multiples. Pregnancy complications from a multiple pregnancy may increase the risk of learning disabilities.

But spotting a learning disability early means your child will get help, gain confidence, and do better in school.

Call your doctor if your child struggles with learning. Watch for the following signs, although experiencing them doesn't necessarily mean your child has a disability. They're red flags to mention to your doctor.

Preschool age: Difficulty learning letters, numbers, colors, shapes, and days of the week; trouble pronouncing words

Find a Gym That Offers Child Care

We joined a gym with child care, and those one or two kid-free hours are amazing! They even have an area for computer work, so I can work out and get some charting done without babies grabbing all my limbs.

—Megan Lemay, MD, a mom of a three-year-old son and 22-month-old twin boys and an assistant professor of internal medicine at the Virginia Commonwealth University School of Medicine, in Richmond

correctly or rhyming words; struggling to find the right word; trouble holding and using crayons, pencils, and scissors; doesn't color in the lines; struggling with buttons, zippers, and snaps; difficulty following directions.

Ages 5 to 9: Trouble linking sounds with letters and blending sounds to make words; getting basic words wrong when reading; taking longer to learn new skills; spells words wrong; difficulty remembering sequences, learning basic math, and telling time.

Ages 10 to 13: Struggling with reading comprehension, math, and word problems; spelling the same word differently on the same page; disliking reading or writing; disorganized room and desk; messy handwriting; struggling to follow discussions and express thoughts.

Homework with twins is a challenge. Inevitably one twin needs help with something and needs more attention than the other. The other one hovers around while I try to explain. I often have to put my foot down and say, "Please go into another room!" I help one twin with his or her homework, then switch to the other.

—*Jennifer Gilbert, DO*

∽

One thing I have done to help my kids with school is to do some extra prep during the summer. I ask my mom friends who have kids a few years older, "What's a big thing they learn next year?" Then we work on that. One year, for example, they learned all of the state capitals.

—*Jennifer Gilbert, DO*

∽

We find it hard to get someone to watch all three kids (age three and under) at bedtime, so we end up getting babysitters for after they go to sleep. Then we go out once they're down.

—*Megan Lemay, MD, a mom of a three-year-old son and 22-month-old twin boys and an assistant professor of internal medicine at the Virginia Commonwealth University School of Medicine, in Richmond*

∽

Having twins really does get easier. I found it got a lot easier when my twins went to kindergarten.

There are many benefits to having twins. It's fun to see them interact. Their closeness is really special.

—*Amy J. Lynch, DO*

Both of my kids like to do activities. It can make for a crazy schedule, but we make it work. I try to encourage them to participate in opposite sports. For example, if one does a fall sport, the other can do something in the winter.

—*Jennifer Gilbert, DO*

Dr. Sonal's Tips

A major challenge in parenting, especially with twins, is making time for you. The best way for me to do this was to exercise. I joined a gym early on. It was a lifesaver. In the beginning, I went only one time a week, but that was better than no times a week! I love to dance, so I took Zumba and Bollywood classes. Having a scheduled class helped me to be committed to going. Going to the gym gave me my own time, helped me get back into shape, and made me feel better about myself.

Another way I make time for myself is by keeping a book on my nightstand. I try to go to bed 20 minutes early so I can read before falling asleep. I started to do this when my girls were around two years old. It has been fantastic.

I also joined a mommy book club, which helps me. I love to read, so it's gotten me back into a hobby. And it's great socializing with other mothers once a month.

Join a Walking Group

Now that the kids are off at school during the day, you hopefully have a few daytime hours for yourself. A great way to get out, socialize, and improve your physical and mental health is to connect with a walking group. Going for brisk walks on a regular basis helps you maintain a healthy weight and lowers your risk for diseases such as heart disease. Some camaraderie with other moms and time to chat will also do wonders for your mood.

Look for other moms to join you on a walking trail or find a walking club online by going to **MEETUP.COM**.

Fast Facts

Kathy Dolan led the effort to create the Twins Law. The Twins Law refers to a law that allows parents of twins or multiples to decide whether or not to place their children in the same classroom. In the past, many schools required mandatory separation of twins and multiples in the classroom even though most psychologists and parents disagreed with that decision. Kathy needed a doctor's note to keep her sons together in kindergarten. After her battle, she founded the Twins Law to push for legislation in every state similar to the Minnesota Statute. Six states—Florida, Georgia, Louisiana, Minnesota, New Hampshire, and Texas—have passed laws allowing parents to keep children together in classrooms.

Mommy MD Guides-Recommended Product
PreparaKit Take Along First Aid Kit

A must-have for every mom and dad, this first aid kit has everything you need for kid-related emergencies in a compact pouch that is just right for purses and bags. The kit includes bandages and ointments from well-known brands to fix everything from scrapes and bruises to bug bites. You'll find them for around $19.97 at **AMAZON.COM**.

Chapter 9:

Outings, Day Trips, and Vacations

It's harder for moms of multiples to get out of the house. Even the basics—getting multiples into the car safely when you're alone—can be a logistical puzzle. But getting out for some fresh air or to run errands is important for you and your babies.

Moms of multiples rely on double or triple strollers, a double wearable baby carrier, or carry one baby while the other is in a carrier to get around with their babies. And keep in mind that the distractions of getting more than one baby in and out of the car can make it too easy to lock your keys inside. With that in mind, always crack at least one window before putting your babies in their car seats (or get in the habit of leaving a front seat door open) and have an extra set of car keys in your wallet, house, or key hider near your front door.

Packing as light as possible will save your back, but you want to make sure have everything you need. If you're out just for a few hours, pack at least a few diapers for each kid, wipes, a portable changing pad, bottles and formula or a nursing cover, bibs, burp cloths, Ziploc bags for dirty clothes, hand sanitizer, at least one set of clothes per baby, and pacifiers. Plus, don't forget your own necessities, such as your wallet and phone. You might also want to keep a diaper bag in your car with extra diapers, wipes, water, and a first aid kit.

If you're going on a day trip, you'll also need enough diapers and formula to get through the day, your breast pump if you're still pumping, water, snacks and baby food and utensils if your babies are old enough for solids, extra shirts for you if your babies tend to spit up, and a first aid kit with Band-Aids and antibiotic ointment.

For vacations, you'll need all of that plus car seats to bring on the plane if you're flying, a double or triple umbrella stroller that folds easily, medications (acetaminophen or ibuprofen in case a baby gets sick), baby shampoo and baby wash, toys, books, a Pack 'n Play, extra blankets, and a white noise machine (or use a white noise app on your phone). Also be sure to have your passports and babies' birth certificates if you're traveling internationally.

Fast Facts

Formula and breast milk for infants is permitted by the TSA in containers smaller than 3.4 ounces. Check the TSA website, TSA.gov, before traveling for updates to their requirements.

When my twins were two weeks old, I started getting out for walks. I would "wear" them or use the double city mini-stroller.

My advice is to get a stroller and get out every single day. You feel like a milk cow and you're so tired, but you need to get outside. The worst that can happen is they scream. It's not the end of the world! I think my twins did so well because we went out so often.

—*Cassie Cole, MD, a mom of five-year-old twin girls and an emergency physician, in Hot Springs, AR*

DR. SONAL'S TIPS

After our twins' first few months, my husband and I were getting "cabin fever" from being in the house all of the time. We started taking the girls on walks around the neighborhood. My husband and I each donned a baby carrier, and we each "wore" a girl on our walks. The walks got us out of the house, and we got some exercise. Our girls enjoyed them too.

When our girls got too heavy to carry, we transitioned to using a stroller. I wish I had chosen a lighter stroller. We didn't want to use a side-by-side stroller because it was too wide, so we chose a front-and-back stroller. The car seats clipped in, which was convenient. But the whole getup was just too heavy.

DR. SONAL'S TIPS

How and when you take your twins out will depend on your comfort level. Initially, when my girls were little, we didn't get out much. Our first big outing was when the girls were two and a half months old, and my sister was having a New Year's Eve party at her house. I felt comfortable because we were at my sister's house, and there would be multiple people to help.

The first time I took them out alone was when they were four months old. A mother from our twins' mom group was having a playdate at her house. She was extremely helpful, and it felt good to be out and to talk to other mothers and not feel like I was so alone. I highly recommend joining a local or online twins mom group.

Grocery shopping with twins is an adventure. Only a few stores have the carts for multiple children, such as Target and Costco. I shopped there a lot for that reason.

—Brooke A. Jackson, MD, a mom of 11-year-old twin girls and a 9-year-old son, a dermatologist, and the founder and medical director of the Skin Wellness Dermatology Associates, in Durham, NC

Fast Facts

A study published in 1971 found that twins had a higher chance of having car sickness. Car sickness is roughly five times more frequent in twins when one or both parents experienced car sickness as children.

Early on with our twins, even going to the grocery store was a family affair. My husband and I would both go. One of us would push a cart with the babies; the other would push a cart with the groceries.

> —*Amy J. Lynch, DO, a mom of eight-year-old twin boys and a five-year-old son and a physical medicine and rehabilitation specialist at the Iowa Clinic, in Des Moines*

DR. SONAL'S TIPS

Of course, we had to take our girls on plenty of errands in the car. I learned it is helpful to think about your car choice ahead of time. We did not buy a minivan until the girls were a year old. I wish we would have gotten it sooner. My husband and I both had big sedans, but it was a pain getting a large double stroller in and out of the trunk and constantly having to bend down to put the car seats in. The minivan made life much easier.

Here are some other items I often keep in my car:

- *Extra diapers: I always kept extra diapers in there. If you forget your diaper bag at home, having extra diapers and wipes in the car helps.*
- *Extra clothes: I started storing extra clothes in the car as well. One time we were out on a walk at the park and there was a diaper leak with poop everywhere. The extra clothes came in very handy!*
- *Extra blankets: Having a bigger vehicle also lets you store a couple of extra blankets in the car. This is invaluable*

when the weather changes, if your clothes get wet, or if a diaper leaks. When all else fails, at least you have some blankets.

- Baby wipes: When my girls were younger, I kept diaper wipes in my car. Now that they're older, I store wet wipes for their hands and sanitizing wipes to clean up spills.
- Hand sanitizer
- Towel: A towel is handy to wipe up a spill or if somebody gets wet.
- Nonperishable snacks
- Plastic bags: You never know when you'll have wet clothes or something you need to put in there.
- Sunscreen
- Band-Aids in a small first aid kit
- Tools or a small road emergency kit with cable jumpers and a flashlight
- Things to do: I usually have a clipboard and coloring books, or some sort of activity book for them in the car. We spend a lot of time in the car, and I don't like them to always be watching a DVD. We do have a DVD player in the car. I also always have lots of music in the car for when they want to sing or listen to music.
- Activity backpacks: For when we went to restaurants, I had special "restaurant backpacks" for them. I stocked them with things they didn't normally play with, so they were novelties to them, such as puzzles or mini blocks. That

Find a Babysitter You Trust

I don't think I'm doing a great job of taking time for myself. It's something I really need to work on. I do go out to dinner occasionally with girlfriends, and my husband and I have gone on a couple of dates since the boys were born, but we need to do this more often. We do have a good group of babysitters we have found and like, so we feel very comfortable leaving them. But when we're not working, we usually just enjoy family time.

—Andrea Orr, MD, a mom of 10-month-old twin boys
and a pediatrician with Northwest Pediatrics
Washington University Clinical Associates, in St. Louis, MO

would occupy the twins for a while, and we could have a quieter meal.

∽

When we took our twins on a trip, such as out of town to visit family, we got the car all packed. Then we fed the twins, got them into their car seats, and went. This gave us around four hours to drive, which coincidentally is about the distance to drive home to our families. By the time we got there, we had two screaming babies. We'd give them a quick bottle, and then they were fine.

—*Amy J. Lynch, DO*

DR. SONAL'S TIPS

A trick that I didn't actually use but wish I had was keeping an extra training potty lined with a diaper in the back of the minivan. When a toddler is learning to toilet train, sometimes she has to go in a hurry. You can't always quickly find a public restroom to stop at.

❦

We made traveling with the twins easier by using lots of extra hands! We usually recruited a family member to travel with us when we could.

—*Anne Rodrigue, DO, a mom of two-year-old twin girls and an ob-gyn at Thibodaux Women's Center, in Louisiana*

❦

I learned you can rent double strollers from companies who will deliver to your destination prior to your arrival. That's a lifesaver!

—*Saira Butt, MD, a mom of three-year-old twins and an infectious diseases physician, in Carmel, IN*

❦

Traveling is huge. I find it interesting that there's always some woman on the plane who will hold a stranger's child while the husband happily drinks coffee.

To this day, if I see a mom traveling alone, I will offer to help carry her bag.

—*Brooke A. Jackson, MD*

Accept the fact that travel with kids is going to take you extra time and make sure you plan for it. Arrive way ahead of the airport's recommended minimum time before flights, for example. Bring lots of snacks, 10 more diapers, an extra pack of wipes, and two more changes of clothes than you think you will need.

—*Anne Rodrigue, DO*

With twins, more is more! Always have more diapers than you think you'll need, more wipes than you think you'll need, and more extra pairs of clothes than you think you'll need. Trust me, you'll need them! Though I'm sure long-distance travel is possible, we chose to avoid any major trips in the first year due to how difficult it would be with three children under the age of four.

—*Meredith Brauer, MD, a mom of a three-year-old daughter and six-month-old boy-girl twins and an internal medicine hospitalist at Central DuPage Hospital, in Winfield, IL*

When we travel, we always bring our kids' car seats. In order to get the car seats through the terminal, practice before you get there by strapping the car seats to the back of your double stroller. You can push the kids through the airport and won't break your back trying to carry the seats.

—*Valerie Sheppard, MD, a mom of 5-year-old boy/girl twins and a pediatrician with Newport Children's Medical Group, in Newport Beach, CA*

We took the boys on their first flight when they were almost six months old. We gave ourselves more time than we needed, and it wasn't at all stressful.

The best move we made was that we talked about our plan ahead of time and what each of our jobs was going to be. We gate-checked two car seats and their stroller and timed their bottles with takeoff and landing.

—*Andrea Orr, MD, MD, a mom of 10-month-old twin boys and a pediatrician with Northwest Pediatrics Washington University Clinical Associates, in St. Louis, MO*

❧

Don't be afraid to ask for help—especially if you're traveling alone. I asked the airline to help me get my twins' car seats onto the plane, so I could just worry about getting the twins out of their stroller and down the aisle when I was traveling solo.

Also, check all your baggage except your diaper bag—you just won't have free hands for any carry-ons.

—*Valerie Sheppard, MD*

❧

If possible, we try to plan travel times so the twins can still have their normal night's sleep, naps, feeding times, and other scheduled activities. Unfortunately, this isn't always possible.

—*Anne Rodrigue, DO*

My husband and I flew with our twins when they were five months old. We held them on our laps. It was only a three-hour flight, so it wasn't a big deal.

However, baby carriers for Mom and Dad in the airport are a must!

Now that our twins are nearly two years old, we buy an entire row of seats. We hold them in our laps for takeoffs and landings, and we set them on one seat for the rest of the flight.

—Leah Cobb, MD, a mom of 20-month-old twins and a pediatric orthopedic surgeon at San Jorge Children's Hospital, in San Juan, PR

Fast Facts

When creating or updating your family tree, a genogram can be used to represent a trait within a family tree. These are the symbols indicating identical and fraternal twins within the family chart:

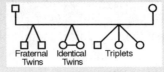

I traveled twice with my twins by myself (at ages two months and 2½ years) and three times together with my husband (at ages nine months, 18 months, and nearly three years old) by plane. Based on those experiences, here are key things to pack:

• For bottle-feeding infants, have bottles ready to go on the plane with the powder already in the bottles. Then, you'll just have to add water rather than trying to measure powder on a bumpy plane ride.

Try to prepare the bottles out of sight and have them ready to use at takeoff and landing to prevent ear discomfort.

• We used car seats during all of our flights, and I highly recommend it. Just as our twins knew they couldn't get out of their car seats in cars, we treated air travel the same and told them that they couldn't get up on the plane.

Even as toddlers, they mostly stayed in their seats without a fuss and fell asleep because their seats felt like a comfortable, familiar environment to them.

• Bring lots and lots of toys and snacks to occupy your toddler twins on the plane. When they were toddlers, we brought new small books, paper and stickers, Tegu blocks, activity books with magic markers, toy cars, stuffed animals, and several zip-lock bags filled with their favorite snacks.

• Finally, bring three or four spare outfits for infant twins, and hopefully you won't experience diaper blowouts and vomit during the same flight like I did once!

—*Valerie Sheppard, MD*

Dr. Sonal's Tips

We took our twins to a hotel for the first time when they were a year old. We requested two cribs ahead of time. There was a balcony, and the hotel staff couldn't guarantee we'd have a first-floor room, so they put mesh around the balcony for parents with small children. If they hadn't put up that mesh, which most hotels probably don't do, we would have made sure we had a room on the first floor. And certainly, we'd have kept the door to the balcony locked. We went back to that hotel several times.

For plane travel, I made up two travel backpacks. I stocked them with some snacks, blankies, coloring books, triangular-shaped crayons, and other things that didn't easily roll off the plane tray tables. These things kept them occupied. The girls did great on the plane even at age four. Another passenger complimented me after the flight on how well-behaved my girls were—without resorting to electronics!

Make sure to bring a small bottle of children's pain reliever, Band-Aids, headache medicine for yourself, and your insurance card. You never know when an emergency might strike, and it is better to be safe than sorry.

Fast Facts

Taking care of twins is very time consuming, and many moms of twins find it difficult to leave their homes. A 2008 survey done by the Twins and Multiple Births Association (TAMBA) found that mothers of multiples are frequently alone, with nearly half of mothers (48 percent) spending less than an hour a day talking to another adult.

We have traveled extensively. We check our babies' car seats, strollers, and carriers at the check-in counter. We check all of our bags—except for the diaper bag.

When traveling, I use a large backpack for a diaper bag. This way, I have both hands free.

When we travel, we bring lots of books for our twins. We don't do screen time, but they love to read books.

—*Leah Cobb, MD*

Set your children's expectations for the flight days before and reinforce them the day you travel. Explain that being on a plane is like being in a restaurant: Use quiet indoor voices, ask politely for things you want, and no crying or screaming.

—*Valerie Sheppard, MD, a mom of 5-year-old boy/girl twins and a pediatrician with Newport Children's Medical Group, in Newport Beach, CA*

Don't forget an extra "support" blanket/paci/lovie. My kids use lovies. In our case, these are small stuffed animals (one is a lamb and one is a cow) made with different fabrics and textures and about the size of a quarter of a swaddle blanket.

We bring these on the plane or car ride, even though the twins usually only sleep with them, and we have an extra backup in our carry-ons in case one goes missing or the luggage doesn't arrive. We also take our sound machine with us everywhere.

—*Anne Rodrigue, DO*

When to Call Your Doctor: Scrapes and Bruises

Little knees get scraped and elbows get bruised. It's all part of growing up. Most of the time a scrape needs to be cleaned and covered with a bandage (with a dab of antibiotic ointment) and a bruise needs a kiss (plus elevation and ice wrapped in a towel if it's severe).

Incidents that require a doctor's care include scrapes that are large and need stitches, contain dirt or gravel, are draining, or are red or swollen. Call a doctor for a bruise if it's painful and swollen or if there's a lump over the bruise.

We don't travel! Mostly I'm joking, but in truth, we really haven't been traveling long distances lately. Luckily, most of our family lives close to us. A well-packed diaper bag is absolutely key for any trips, long or short! One key to this is not to overpack. I recommend diapers (two more than you think you need), a change of clothes for each child, a small pack of wipes, a small blanket, snacks, and a change of shirt for you. I also keep a crate of toys behind the front seat of the car so I can hand one back to them in their seats when they get fussy.

—*Megan Lemay, MD, a mom of a three-year-old son and 22-month-old twin boys and an assistant professor of internal medicine at the Virginia Commonwealth University School of Medicine, in Richmond*

On-the-Go Safety Checklist

- Create a list of any allergies and medical conditions your babies have and store it with their insurance cards in your wallet.
- Keep a current photo of your babies in your wallet.
- Give an allergy list, insurance card, and photo to your partner as well.
- Dress your babies in one layer more than you wear.
- Keep your babies out of the sun.
- Put on sunscreen 20 to 30 minutes before going outside.
- Protect your babies' eyes with sunglasses.
- Choose a baby carrier with a back that's deep enough to support them well.
- Consider a stroller with large wheels and a heavy-duty suspension.
- Buy a stroller with a five-point harness.

- Always buckle the safety harness.
- Don't overload the stroller with bags, which could cause it to become off balance.
- Be on the lookout for choking hazards; use a toilet paper tube as a guide. (Anything that fits

Mommy MD Guides–Recommended Products for Twins Travel

Joovy Scooter X2 Double Stroller

When you are expecting multiples, you face an endless list of things to prepare. Perhaps you won't even think about the difficulties of carting a double stroller around crowded streets and stores. That's okay. The people at Joovy have got you covered. Joovy's Scooter X2 Double Stroller will get you, and the kids, through the door! Its lightweight, narrow design lets you breeze through most standard doorways, without any folding. It also has independent reclining adjustable side-by-side seats that hold up to 45 pounds each (90 pounds total). It also boasts the biggest storage basket on the market. It retails for $209.99 at AMAZON.COM.

Prince Lionheart Stroller Connectors

Smart. Easy. These durable molded plastic stroller connectors snap onto a variety of stroller tubes, allowing you to turn two strollers into one. They're easy to remove by squeezing the handle. You can purchase them for about $19.97 at AMAZON.COM.

inside the tube is a potential choking hazard.)

- At your destination, keep an even closer eye on your babies.
- Make a habit to check your babies for ticks at every bath.

Weego Twin Baby Carrier

Another must-have item for moms on the go is the Weego Twin Baby Carrier. The Weego carrier is specially designed for twins from birth (4 pounds and up) to approximately five to six months old. The max weight is 33 pounds.

Because of its special construction, you can put two babies in the Weego Twin carrier quickly and, most importantly, without any help. Then the babies can also be passed to another person without removing them from the carrier. The Weego Twin carrier features a unique double-pouch system that ensures the orthopedically correct posture of your babies.

Weegos are machine washable and run about $169.00. You can get them at **WEEGO.COM**.

Baby Trend Universal Double Snap-N-Go Stroller Frame

For transporting two infants in car seats, the Baby Trend Universal Double Snap-N-Go is the way to go. It allows parents to easily place car seats onto the carriage frame without having to remove the child from the carrier. It comes with a two-cup holder and a covered storage container for Mom and Dad. To make things even easier, it folds conveniently with one hand. Find it at **AMAZON.COM** for around $79.99.

Use an Online Personal Stylist

You're venturing out into the world with your babies, and you need to look cute! You *could* rummage through your closet for something to wear, but after you've given birth and been in the thick of things taking care of multiples, your old skinny jeans may not look all that appealing.

It's time for a new outfit, but how do you fit a double stroller into a dressing room? No problem—when the dressing room is your very own bedroom.

When you sign up for an online personal stylist such as Stitch Fix, you'll have clothes shipped directly to you at home. You can try them on at your convenience and return anything you don't like. You'll pay a styling fee up front that will be applied to any clothes you decide to keep. Even better, you can order boxes of clothes whenever you want. Plus, there are plenty of services to choose from, including Stitch Fix, Trunk Club by Nordstrom, and Dia & Co. (which is specifically for plus sizes). Just be sure to read their websites before signing up to be certain you agree with their prices and terms.

Join a Mothers of Twins Club

It's a sad fact that parents of multiples tend to feel isolated and alone. That's why it's so important to connect with others, especially those who know exactly what you're going through. Multiples of America helps parents connect through local clubs that provide networking, information, and get-togethers with other parents of multiples. As a member, you'll also be invited to their Facebook page, where you can interact with other parents online. The membership dues are only $10 a year. If there's not a club in your area, Multiples of America will help you organize one. Find out more about this organization at **MULTIPLES OFAMERICA.ORG**.

Take an Hour (or Two) for Yourself on Vacation

Traveling with multiples is an adventure. An adventure that requires multiple car seats, profuse amounts of sunscreen, a suitcase full of swim diapers, and—inevitably—a few meltdowns.

It's only fair that *you* get a little time to enjoy yourself. The perfect time to steal away: naptime. Let your spouse handle the naps in the hotel room while you do something you enjoy, whether it's walking on the beach, strolling through shops, or lying in peace by the pool. The next day, you take naptime duty so your partner can have some fun.

Index

Note: <u>Underlined</u> references indicate boxed text.

A

Acetaminophen, 24, 90, 139
Activities, for outings, 143–44
Adoptive mothers, 37, <u>45</u>
Advice
　to mothers-to-be, 25–26
　to parents of twins, 77–78
Air travel, 139, <u>139</u>, 146–49, 150–51
Allergies, <u>46</u>, 96
Allergy list, 153
Appliance safety, 107
Apps, for tracking feedings and
　diapering, 59
Arguments, 119

B

Baby A and Baby B, location of,
　<u>27</u>
Baby Brezza, 56
Baby carriers, 138, 140, 148, 153
　Weego Twin Baby Carrier, <u>155</u>
Baby gates, 24, 113
Babyproofing, 100–103. *See also*
　Safety checklists
Baby Shusher, 75

Babysitters, 43, <u>88</u>, 134, <u>144</u>.
　See also Nannies
Baby Tracker app, 59
Baby Trend Universal Double
　Snap-N-Go Stroller
　Frame, <u>155</u>
Baby wipes, 61, 62, <u>63</u>, 142, 143,
　146
Backpacks
　as diaper bag, 151
　for outings and travel, 143–44,
　150
Bassinets
　co-sleeping in, 73–74
　The HALO Twin Bassinest, <u>86</u>
Bathing, 82, 83
Bathroom safety checklist, 105–7
Bathtub, baby, 105
Battery storage, 23
Bedroom safety checklist, 111
Bedtime routines. *See* Sleep
　routines
Bilingual language development,
　129
Birthday parties, 115, 117, 118

Birth weight
  low, 18
  of singletons vs. multiples, 21
Blankets, stored in car, 142–43
Book club, 136
Books, 151
Boppy pillow, 44, 49, 53
Bottlefeeding, 42, 43, 46, 53–54
  air travel and, 149
  chart for tracking, 43
  formula for (*see* Formula)
  pillow for, <u>31</u>, 44
Bottle warmers, 56
Bouncer seat safety, 108, 109
Bowel movements, first, 58
Brauer, Meredith, 47–48, 62, <u>65</u>,
    66, 82, 93, 146
Breastfeeding
  chart for tracking, 41, 52
  getting help with, 41–42, 45, 48
  holds for, 41
  pillows for, <u>31</u>, <u>32</u>, 44, 48–49,
    53
  of premature babies, 40–41, 46,
    48–49
  stress about, 47, 52
Breast milk
  benefits of, 40
  producing, for multiples, 41
  TSA allowance for, <u>139</u>
  warming, 56
Breast pump(ing), 41, 45, 46, 48,
    49, <u>51</u>, 54–55, 108
Bronchiolitis, <u>90</u>
Bruises, when to call your doctor
    about, <u>152</u>
Butt, Saira, 19, 42, 61, 66, 75, <u>78</u>,
    145

C
Car
  choosing, 142
  supplies to keep in, 142–44
Carbon monoxide alarms, 23
Carriers. *See* Baby carriers
Car safety, 138
Car seats, 101, 146, 147, 149, 151
  Baby Trend Universal Double
    Snap-N-Go Stroller
    Frame for, <u>155</u>
Car sickness, <u>141</u>
Cesarean section, 19, 32–33, 34
Changing table, 63, 64, 105, 110
Chemicals, safety with, 112, 113
Choking hazards, 23, 109, 154–55
Cleaning products safety, 107
Clothing. *See also* Dressing
  extra, stored in car, 69, 142
  hand-me-down, 67, 72
  quilt made from, 118
  shopping for, 70, 71
  for travel, 146, 149
  washing, 69, 105
Cobb, Leah, 44, 45, 56, 60, 62,
    79, 82, 84, 91, <u>131</u>, 148, 151
Coffee break, <u>124</u>
Colds, 89–90
Cole, Cassie, 29, 49, 62, 66, 68,
    102, 140
Colic, 95
Colostrum, 40
Competition, <u>120</u>
Consumer Product Safety
    Commission, 23
Co-sleeping for multiples, 73–74,
    75, 83
Coupons, diaper, <u>71</u>

Cribs, 74, 75, 83, 84, 86
    safety guidelines for, 104, 105
Crying, 54, 95
Crying it out, for sleep training,
        84–85
Cryptophasia, 39

D

Dairy products, 23
Date nights, 110
Day care, 127, 128
Day trips, 139, 142–44. *See also*
        Travel
Dental health, influences on, 53
Dental records, of identical twins,
        91
Dia & Co., 156
Diaper bag
    for air travel, 147, 151
    stocking, 69, 139, 152
Diaper changes
    locations for, 60, 62–63, 64,
        105, 110
    nighttime, 62, 64, 81–82
    number of, 58, 67, 68, 70
    time spent on, 69
    tracking, 41, 58, 59
Diaper cream, 61, 62
Diaper disposal receptacle, 62
Diaper rash, 61
Diapers
    cost of, 71
    coupons for, 71
    as potty liner, 65, 145
    for travel, 142, 146
    types of, 60, 61, 64
Diapers and Wipes Bundle from
        Honest Company, 63

Dining room safety checklist,
        109–9
Discipline, 118
Dishwasher safety, 107
Dolan, Kathy, 137
Dressing, 66–72. *See also*
        Clothing
    in different outfits, 68, 70, 71
    in matching outfits, 66–67, 68,
        72
Dr. Sonal's Tips
    on breastfeeding vs. bottle
        feeding, 52–55
    on car choice, 142
    on car trip supplies, 142–44
    on colic, 95
    on diapering, 61, 64, 81–82
    on dressing, 67
    on emotions during twin
        pregnancy, 21
    on finding out babies' gender,
        22
    on first-time outings, 141
    on getting help after birth,
        34–35
    on individual treatment of
        twins, 123–24
    on making time for yourself,
        135–36
    on maternity leave, 129
    on monitoring pregnancy's
        progress, 25
    on naming babies, 116
    on one-on-one time, 120
    on outdoor walks with babies,
        140
    on pacifiers, 97
    on potty training, 65, 145

Dr. Sonal's Tips *(cont.)*
  on prenatal nutrition, 22
  on returning to work, 129
  on separating twins at school,
    130
  on sleep, 76, 83
  on strangers' comments about
    pregnancy, 26
  on travel, 145, 150
  on unsolicited advice, 26
  on visitors, 99

E

Eat Sleep Poop app, 59
Eczema, 97, 124
Electrical outlet covers, 105, 111
Electrical safety, 107, 108, 110, 112
Elliot, Amy Ann, <u>38</u>
Elliot, Kate Marie, <u>38</u>
Emergency phone numbers, 22,
    100–101
Emotions
  during pregnancy, 17, 20, 21
  after preterm delivery, 27
Extrasensory perception (ESP), <u>120</u>

F

Falls
  consolation for, 102
  preventing, 24
  when to call your doctor about,
    <u>101</u>
Family tree, <u>148</u>
Fatigue. *See also* Sleep deprivation
  first-trimester, 18, <u>25</u>
Feeding. *See* Bottlefeeding;
    Breastfeeding
Feeding charts, 41, 43, 52, 59

Feeding help, 42, 43
Feeding schedule, 42, 43, 45, 51
Feeding set, <u>47</u>
Feeding station, 42
Fertilization, 17–18
Fevers, <u>54</u>, 90
Fireplace safety, 111
Fire safety, 22–23
First aid class, 22
First aid kit, 24, <u>137</u>
Fisher-Price Rock 'n Play Sleeper,
    <u>87</u>
Flores, Cassandra, <u>38</u>
Flores, Isaiah, <u>38</u>
Flores, Israel, <u>38</u>
Flu vaccine, 90
Formula
  in Organic Formula Bundle
    Packs, <u>63</u>
  safety with, 108
  TSA allowance for, <u>139</u>
Formula feeding, 42, 43, 47, 48,
    50, 51, 52–53, 54
Fraternal twins
  allergies of, <u>46</u>
  blood types of, <u>39</u>
  dairy products increasing
    chance of, <u>23</u>
  gender of, <u>31</u>
  genogram for, <u>148</u>
  pregnancy risk with, <u>34</u>
  survival rates of, <u>119</u>
  twin births among, <u>20</u>
Friends, shared vs. separate, 132
Furniture anchors, 100, <u>103</u>, 105,
    108, 110
Furniture hazards, removing, 111,
    113

G

Garage safety checklist, 112

Gemellology (study of twins), 129

Gender of babies, finding out, 19, 21, 22

Genogram, on family tree, 148

Gilbert, Jennifer, 19, 42, 70, 117, 119, 120, 121, 130, 134, 135

Grocery shopping, 141–42

Ground fault circuit interrupters, 107, 108

Gym
with child care, 133
joining, 135–36
safety checklist for, 112

H

Half-identical twins, 29

HALO Twin Bassinest, The, 86

Hand washing, 89, 108, 109

Hatch Baby changing pad, 59

Head injury, when to call your doctor about, 101

Health challenges, managing, 89–99

Healthy Sleep Habits, Happy Child, 85

Heather's Tips
on enjoying twins, 131
on good online advice, 77–78
on helping others identify your twins, 126
on organizing toys, 103
on premature babies in NICU, 27

HELLP syndrome, 32

Helpers. *See also* Babysitters; Nannies
after bringing babies home, 34–35, 37

family visitors as, 99
for feeding, 42, 43
at nighttime, 76

High blood pressure
with preeclampsia, 32, 33
during pregnancy, 18

High chair, 109

Homework, 134

Honest Company products, 63

Hotel safety, 150

Hyperovulation gene, 38

I

Ibuprofen, 90, 139

Identical twins
allergies of, 46
with different hair and eye color, 39
dogs identifying, 117
fingerprints of, 39
gender of, 31
genogram for, 148
heights and weights of, 33
higher-risk pregnancy with, 34
incidence of, 37
survival rates of, 119
teeth of, 91
Twin to Twin Transfusion Syndrome in, 28
voices of, 98

Identification of twins, 126

Illnesses
managing, 89–90
preventing, 90
when to call your doctor about, 54–55

Individuality, fostering, 114–26

Infant CPR class, 22

J

Jackson, Brooke A., 25, 37, 43, 44, 45, <u>45</u>, 68, 80, 81, 85, 87, 96, 98, 117, 118, 119, 121, 141, 145

Jones-Elliot, Maria, <u>38</u>

Joovy Scooter X2 Double Stroller, <u>154</u>

Journaling about milestones, 117

Juvenile Products Manufacturers Association (JPMA) seal, 23, 104

K

Karpinsky, Heather, 14–15, <u>47</u>. *See also* Heather's Tips

Kindness, modeling, 121

Kitchen safety checklist, 107–8

L

Labels, from NameBubbles, <u>125</u>

Labor, premature, when to call your doctor about, <u>30</u>

Lactation consultants, 42, 48, 52

Lead exposure, 24

Learning disability, when to call your doctor about, <u>132–33</u>

Left-handedness, 118, <u>128</u>

Lemay, Megan, 48–49, 60, 66, 81, 94, <u>133</u>, 134, 152

Living room safety checklist, 109–11

Loneliness, of mothers of twins, <u>150</u>

Longevity
of mothers of twins, <u>37</u>
of twins vs. singletons, <u>119</u>

Lovies, 151

Low birth weight, 18

Lynch, Amy J., 20, 21, 32–33, 35, 36, 37, 43, 51, 60, 67, 69, 71, 77, 84, 86, 95, 122, 132, 134, 142, 144

M

Massage, prenatal, <u>36</u>

Maternity leave, 37, 80, 129

Medication
safety with, 106
for travel, 139, 150

Milestone Original Baby Photo Cards, <u>122</u>

Milestones
journaling about, 117
missed, when to call your doctor about, <u>99</u>

Minivan, 142

Mirror image twins, <u>39</u>

Mommy MD Guides– Recommended Products

Baby Trend Universal Double Snap-N-Go Stroller Frame, <u>155</u>

Diapers and Wipes Bundle from Honest Company, <u>63</u>

Fisher-Price Rock 'n Play Sleeper, <u>87</u>

The HALO Twin Bassinest, <u>86</u>

Joovy Scooter X2 Double Stroller, <u>154</u>

Milestone Original Baby Photo Cards, <u>122</u>

My Brest Friend Twin Plus Breastfeeding Pillow, <u>32</u>

NameBubbles.com, <u>125</u>

Nokire TV Strap Anti-Tip Child Safety Furniture Straps, 103
PreparaKit Take Along First Aid Kit, 137
Prince Lionheart Stroller Connectors, 154
Pure Spoon, 50
RealKidShades.com, 135
The Twin Feeding Set from BabyA-BabyB.com, 47
Twin Z Pillow, 31
Weego Twin Baby Carrier, 155
YUP Extra-Large Stroller Hooks, 153
MomMy Time
  celebrating the end of pumping, 51
  coffee break and reading time, 124
  date nights, 110
  finding a babysitter, 144
  hiring a part-time nanny, 131
  joining a gym with child care, 133
  joining a mothers of twins club, 156–57
  joining a walking group, 136
  letting chores slide, 65
  movie watching, 57
  napping, 88
  Pilates, 113
  prenatal spa treatment, 36
  running, 45
  taking advantage of early bedtime, 78
  using an online personal stylist, 156
  on vacations, 157

Mothers of twins clubs, 141, 156–57
Mouth bacteria, 53
Movies, recommended, 57
Multiple pregnancy
  challenges during, 18, 25
  emotions during, 17, 20, 21
  finding out about, 19, 20, 21
  higher risk with, 34
  nutrition during, 18, 22
  self-care during, 18
  strangers' comments about, 26
Multiples. See also Quadruplets; Triplets; Twins
  conception of, 17–18
  delivery of, 19, 32–33
Multiples of America, 157
My Brest Friend Twin Plus Breastfeeding Pillow, 32, 49

N

NameBubbles.com, 125
Names, choosing, 36, 116
Nannies, 51, 65, 85, 102, 129. See also Babysitters
  nighttime, 35, 79–80
  part-time, 131
Napping, 76, 81, 88, 157. See also Sleep
Nausea, first-trimester, 18
NICU, premature babies in, 27, 29, 48, 92–93
Night-light, 105, 111
Nighttime waking, when to call your doctor about, 75
Noise, coping with, 113

Nokire TV Strap Anti-Tip Child
    Safety Furniture Straps, <u>103</u>
Nursery safety checklist, 104–5
Nutrition, prenatal, 18, 22

O

Office safety checklist, 111
One-on-one time with twins,
    120, 121, 122
Online personal stylist, <u>156</u>
On-the-go safety checklist, 153–55
Organic Formula Bundle Packs, <u>63</u>
Orr, Andrea, 44, 50, 63, 66, 74,
    76, 83, 92, 94, <u>144</u>, 147
Outings. *See also* Travel
    difficulty of, 138
    first-time, 141
    grocery shopping, 141–42
    outdoor walks, 140
    packing for, 138–39, 142–44
Oxygen, supplemental, 94

P

Pacifiers, 84, 97
Packing, for travel, 138–39
Pajamas, 66, 104
Pampers Swaddlers diapers, 60
Patel, Sonal R., 13. *See also* Dr.
    Sonal's Tips
Personality, fostering, 114–26
Personality traits, inherited, <u>121</u>
Personal stylist, online, <u>156</u>
Peters, Maria, 45, 72, <u>113</u>
Phone numbers, emergency, 22,
    100–101
Pilates, <u>113</u>
Pillows, for breastfeeding, <u>31</u>, <u>32</u>,
    44, 48–49, 53

Plants, safety with, 111, 113
Positive reinforcement, 119
Potty training, 65, 145
Preeclampsia, symptoms of, 32, 33
Pregnancy. *See* Multiple pregnancy
Premature babies
    breastfeeding, 40–41, 46, 48–49
    in NICU, 27, 29, 48, 92–93
Premature labor, when to call
    your doctor about, <u>30</u>
Prenatal spa treatment, <u>36</u>
PreparaKit Take Along First Aid
    Kit, <u>137</u>
Preterm delivery
    emotions after, 27
    worries about, 18, 21, 26
Prince Lionheart Stroller
    Connectors, <u>154</u>
Product safety, 23
Pure Spoon foods, <u>50</u>

Q

Quadruplets
    average birth weight of, <u>21</u>
    premature birth of, 18
Quilt, made from clothing, 118

R

Rahman, Hiba, <u>39</u>
Rahman, Rumasia, <u>39</u>
Reading, <u>124</u>, 136
Real Kids Shades, for eye
    protection, <u>135</u>
Reflux, 95
Respiratory syncytial virus
    (RSV), <u>90</u>
Restaurants, activity backpacks
    for, 143–44

Rockers/rocking, 45, 81, <u>87</u>

Rodrigue, Anne, 42, 44, 56, 61, 68, 84, 97, 145, 146, 147, 151

Rooming in, 34, 35

Running, <u>45</u>

S

Safety, general guidelines for, 100–103

Safety checklists
bathroom, 105–7
bedroom/office, 111
dining room, 108–9
garage/workshop/gym, 112
kitchen, 107–8
living room, 109–11
nursery, 104–5
on-the-go, 153–55
preparing for baby, 22–24
yard, 112–13

School, keeping twins apart or separate in, 128, 130, 132, <u>137</u>

Schoolwork, 134

Scrapes, when to call your doctor about, <u>152</u>

Secret language of twins, <u>39</u>

Self-care, prenatal, 18

Sense of humor, parental, 96

Separation anxiety
in school, 130
when to call your doctor about, <u>123</u>

Sharing, 119

Sheppard, Valerie, 46, <u>51</u>, 60, 62, 69, 79, 84, 92, 146, 147, 149, 151

Sleep. *See also* Napping
co-sleeping for multiples, 73–74, 75, 83
importance of, <u>65</u>, <u>113</u>
nighttime waking and, <u>75</u>
rocking for, 81, 82, <u>87</u>
in same or separate rooms, 86–87

Sleep apnea, <u>75</u>

Sleep deprivation, 76, <u>80</u>, <u>88</u>

Sleep routines, 74, 76, 82–83

Sleep schedules, 73, 77, 79

Sleep training, 84–85

Smoke-free home, 24

Snoring, 96

Solid foods, introducing, 49, <u>50</u>, 56

Spa treatment, prenatal, <u>36</u>

Sports activities, 135

Stitch Fix, <u>156</u>

Stove safety, 107

Stroller Frame, Baby Trend Universal Double Snap-N-Go, <u>155</u>

Strollers, 138, 139, 140
Joovy Scooter X2 Double Stroller, <u>154</u>
Prince Lionheart Stroller Connectors for, <u>154</u>
renting, for trips, 145
safety with, 112, 153–55
YUP Extra-Large Stroller Hooks for, <u>153</u>

Stuffy nose, 90

Sunglasses, 112, <u>135</u>, 153

Sunscreen, 112, 153

Surprise toy boxes, 103

Swaddling, 74

T

Teething, 85, <u>91</u>
Ticks, 155
Toilet lock, 106
Tonsillectomy, 96
Toys
  for air travel, 149
  for car travel, 152
  organizing, 103
  safety with, 105
Travel. *See also* Outings
  alone time during, <u>157</u>
  general tips for, 144–45
  packing for, 138–39, 142–44,
    149, 150, 152
  plane, 139, <u>139</u>, 146–49,
    150–51
  safety tips for, 150, 153–55
  TSA rules for, <u>139</u>
Triplets
  average birth weight of, <u>21</u>
  conception of, 17
  co-sleeping, 74
  diaper changes for, 58
  genogram for, <u>148</u>
  premature birth of, 18
  statistics on, <u>35</u>
Trunk Club by Nordstrom, <u>156</u>
TSA rules, <u>139</u>
TTTS. *See* Twin to Twin
    Transfusion Syndrome
TV anti-tip straps, <u>103</u>
*Twelve Hours' Sleep by Twelve
    Weeks Old*, 84
Twin delivery intervals, <u>38</u>
Twin Feeding Set from
    BabyA-BabyB.com, The,
    <u>47</u>

Twins. *See also* Fraternal twins;
    Identical twins
  healthier mothers having, <u>30</u>
  interacting in womb, <u>19</u>
Twins Law, <u>137</u>
Twin to Twin Transfusion
    Syndrome (TTTS), <u>28</u>,
    <u>34</u>, 91
Twin Z Pillow, <u>31</u>, 44, 48, 49, 60

U

Ultrasound, confirming twin
    pregnancy, 19, 20, 21

V

Vacations. *See* Travel
Vaginal delivery, 19, 32, 33
Viruses, <u>90</u>, 98
Visitors, 99
Voices, of identical twins, <u>98</u>

W

Walking group, joining, <u>136</u>
Walks, with babies, 140
Water temperature control, 105, 106
Weego Twin Baby Carrier, <u>155</u>
Weight gain, of babies, 52
White noise machine, 83
Window treatment safety, 108,
    109, 111
Wipes. *See* Baby wipes
Wipe warmer, 61, 64
Work, returning to, 127, 128, 129
Workshop safety checklist, 112

Y

Yard safety checklist, 112–13
YUP Extra-Large Stroller Hooks,
    <u>153</u>

Acknowledgments

My mother, father, and sister have been my pillars of strength and support. Their unconditional love helped me through college, medical school, residency, and fellowship. Even through hard times, they made sacrifices so that I could succeed.

To my husband, Sujal, for his support and encouragement of all my endeavors.

To my angels Maya and Sophia for their inspiration and eternal love. —Sonal R. Patel, MD

Thank you to the entire Mommy MD Guides team. Working on this project has been a privilege, and I am so proud of what we have created together. I am very grateful to all the incredible doctors who shared their experiences, tips, and words of wisdom. Your time and input have made this book the ultimate resource for parents of multiples.

I am also grateful to have had the opportunity to work with Sonal R. Patel, MD, and Jennifer Bright Reich. This experience has connected me to so many amazing women, and I am honored to have my tips included in this book.

I would also like to thank my twins. I have heard the saying, "it's the little things that make life worth living," but I never knew how true those words were until I met Gavin and Grant.

Thank you to everyone who made this book possible and to our readers. I hope you enjoy this book. —Heather Karpinsky

HUNTINGTON ASTHMA & ALLERGY CENTER

www.myallergymd.com
(888) 475-7784 Fax

Sonal Patel, M.D.
American Board of Allergy & Immunology

Pasadena Office
301 S. Fair Oaks Ave, Ste 401
Pasadena, CA 91105
(626) 793-6680

Burbank Office
2211 W. Magnolia Blvd, Ste 150
Burbank, CA 91506
(818) 309-8452

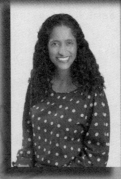

Dr. Patel's
ALLERGY BUSTERS

https://www.facebook.com/Dr-Patels
-Allergy-Busters-126802720686886/

https://www.facebook.com/TMommyMD

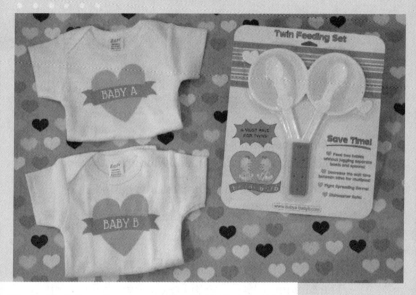

BABY A & BABY B

Baby A & Baby B Gift Set - $25

ALSO BY
MOMOSA PUBLISHING LLC

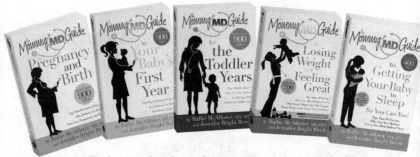

- ● Order our books online at many sites, including Walmart.com, Amazon.com, and MommyMDGuides.com

- ● Purchase them at bookstores nationwide

- ● Download them for your Kindle, Nook, or iPhone/iPad

● ● ●

Enjoy more Mommy MD Guides' tips on

The Mommy MD Guide to Pregnancy and Birth app.

Visit us at MommyMDGuides.com
and DaddyMDGuides.com.

COMING SOON!

*The Mommy MD Guides are hard at work on more titles in the series.
Keep a lookout for:*

The Mommy MD Guide to Keeping Your Baby Safe

About the Authors

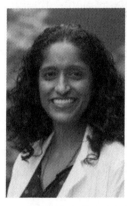

SONAL R. PATEL, MD, MS

Dr. Patel is double board–certified in allergy and clinical immunology as well as pediatrics. She has recently joined Huntington Asthma and Allergy Center in Pasadena, CA. Prior to that, she was with Adventist health for 11 years. She has 20 years of experience working with the underserved.

Dr. Patel initially trained in pediatrics at King-Drew Medical Center in Los Angeles. She then went on to complete a clinical allergy and immunology fellowship at the UCLA School of Medicine. She also completed a Master of Science degree in Clinical Research from Charles R. Drew University of Medicine and Science. Her clinical interests include asthma and atopic dermatitis (eczema).

Dr. Patel has a strong interest in working with inner-city patients and the underserved. She has been on international medical missions to Peru, El Salvador, and Mexico. She has also served on the board for the American Lung Association in California. She is currently on the board of the Los Angeles Society of Allergy, Asthma & Clinical Immunology and the California Society of Allergy, Asthma & Clinical Immunology.

Dr. Patel is a native Angelino. She currently lives in Glendale, California, with her husband and twin daughters. In her spare time she volunteers at her children's elementary school. She is currently learning to knit and crochet. Her other personal interests include traveling, reading, movies, and dance.

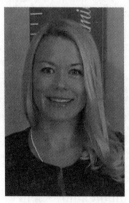

HEATHER STOECKEL KARPINSKY is the founder of Baby A & Baby B LLC and the inventor of the Twin Feeding Set. Heather graduated from Albright College in 2002 and started working for MBNA, a bank based in Wilmington, DE. She took a position in customer service that taught her to "think of yourself as a customer" and "success is finding a better method."

When MBNA was sold, Heather took a new role in

development at the University of Delaware. She helped raise money for scholarships, programs, and research.

The birth of Heather's twins altered her plans and going back to work was not possible. Her focus was on nurturing and caring for her twins, however part of her missed working. When she discovered how simple changes to the products she already used every day would make parenting twins a little easier, her journey as an entrepreneur began.

Heather's new role has helped her grow personally and professionally while connecting her with parents of twins from around the world. Heather lives with her family in Louisiana. She is a member of the Krewe of Hyacinthians and a volunteer for Oschner Hospital.